Successful Aging Through the Life Span

Intergenerational Issues in Health

May L. Wykle, PhD, RN, FAAN, FGSA, is Dean and Florence Cellar Professor of Nursing at the Frances Payne Bolton School of Nursing at Case Western Reserve University. She is the recent past president of the Honor Society of Nursing, Sigma Theta Tau International. Dr. Wykle is presently serving on the advisory board for the Johnson & Johnson national Campaign for Nursing's Future, which is helping address the current nursing shortage with several initiatives aimed at recruiting new nurses and retaining current nurses. She has been a faculty member at Case Western Reserve University since 1969. Since 1988, she has served as director of the University Center on Aging and Health.

Dean Wykle has received numerous honors and awards, including Case's 1989 John S. Diekhoff Award for Excellence in Graduate Teaching, a merit award from the Cleveland Council of Black Nurses, and the 2000 Gerontological Nursing Research Award from the Gerontological Society of America. In August 2003, she was the recipient of the Lifetime Achievement Award from the National Black Nurses Association. Her most recent book, *Serving Minority Elders in the 21st Century,* earned the *American Journal of Nursing's* Book of the Year Award in 2000.

Peter J. Whitehouse, MD, PhD, is Director of Integrative Studies at Case Western Reserve University, as well as professor of neurology, psychiatry, neuroscience, psychology, nursing, organizational behavior, and biomedical ethics and history. He is the founding president of the Intergenerational School, the world's first-ever public multiage, community school. He is active clinically at University Hospitals of Cleveland Joseph Foley Elder Health Center located at Fairhill Center, where he provides care for individuals with concerns about their cognitive abilities as they age. He has a particular interest in narrative medicine and has developed a number of programs focusing on the value of reading and writing for cognitive vitality. These include a project funded by the National Institutes of Health to examine whether book reading delays cognitive impairment as we age and a multimedia family intervention called electronic remembering therapy.

Diana L. Morris, PhD, RN, FAAN, is an associate professor of nursing and associate director for programming at the University Center on Aging and Health, Case Western Reserve University. She has been an associate professor and an affiliate of the Gerontology Center at the Pennsylvania State University. Dr. Morris teaches adult and older adult mental health and cultural competence, as well as epistemology, theory, and research at the graduate level. She has held appointments as a visiting professor and as an associate professor of nursing at the Department of Nursing Science, University of Zimbabwe, where she taught theory and research in the master's degree program. Dr. Morris's research interests include power and well-being in older adults, mental health in older adults (including ethnic minorities), the well-being of family caregivers in the community, and long-term care.

Successful Aging Through the Life Span

Intergenerational Issues in Health

May L. Wykle, PhD, RN, FAAN, FGSA
Peter J. Whitehouse, MD, PhD
Diana L. Morris, PhD, RN, FAAN
Editors

SP Springer Publishing Company

Springer Publishing Company, Inc.
11 W 42nd Street
New York, NY 10036

Acquisitions Editor: Helvi Gold
Production Editor: Sara Yoo
Cover design by Joanne Honigman

05 06 07 08 09 / 5 4 3 2 1

Library of Congress Cataloging-in-Publication Data

Successful aging through the life span : intergenerational issues in health / May L. Wykle, Peter J. Whitehouse, Diane L. Morris, editors.
    p. ; cm.
  Includes bibliographical references
  ISBN 0-8261-2564-6
  1. Older people—Health and hygiene—United States. 2. Older people—United States—Social conditions. 3. Intergenerational relations—United States. 4. Aging—United States.
  [DNLM: 1. Aging. 2. Caregivers. 3. Health Behavior—Aged.
4. Intergenerational Relations. 5. Social Support. WT 104 S942 2005]
  I. Wykle, May L II. Whitehouse, Peter J. III. Morris, Diane L.

RA564.8.S826 2005
613'.0438—dc22

                                   2004022388

Printed in the United States of America by Maple-Vail Book Manufacturing Group.

Contents

Contributors

Patricia A. Adler, PhD(c), RN, CS
Frances Payne Bolton School
  of Nursing
Case Western Reserve University
Cleveland, OH

Tanetta E. Andersson, BA
Doctoral Student
Department of Sociology
Case Western Reserve University
Cleveland, OH

Alexandra Bohne, BA
Doctoral Student
Department of Sociology
Case Western Reserve University
Cleveland, OH

Cameron J. Camp, PhD
Myers Research Institute of
  the Menorah Park Center
  for Senior Living
Beachwood, OH

Amy Dan, MA
Doctoral Student
Department of Sociology
Case Western Reserve University
Cleveland, OH

Peter A. DeGolia, MD, MS
Assistant Professor
Department of Family
  Medicine
School of Medicine
Case Western Reserve University
Cleveland, OH

Stephanie J. FallCreek, DSW
Chief Executive Officer
Fairhill Center
Cleveland, OH

Katherine S. Judge, PhD
The Margaret Blenkner
  Research Institute of
  Benjamin Rose
Cleveland, OH

Eric T. Juengst, PhD
Associate Professor of Bioethics
School of Medicine
Case Western Reserve University
Cleveland, OH

Boaz Kahana, PhD
Professor
Department of Psychology
Cleveland State University
Cleveland, OH

Eva Kahana, PhD
Pierce T. & Elizabeth Robson
   Professor of Humanities
Chair, Department of Sociology
Director, Elderly Care Research
   Center
Case Western Reserve University
Cleveland, OH

Kyle Kercher, PhD
Associate Professor
Department of Sociology
Case Western Reserve University
Cleveland, OH

Jeounghee Kim, MSW
PhD Student
George Warren Brown School
   of Social Work
Washington University
St. Louis, MO

Cathie King, PhD
Project Director
Elderly Care Research Center
Case Western Reserve University
Cleveland, OH

Carolyn Lechner, MSSA
Doctoral Student
Department of Sociology
Case Western Reserve University
Cleveland, OH

Michelle M. Lee, PhD
Myers Research Institute of
   the Menorah Park Center
   for Senior Living
Department of Psychology
Case Western Reserve University
Cleveland, OH

MiJin Lee, MA
PhD Student
George Warren Brown School
   of Social Work
Washington University
St. Louis, MO

Heather Menne, MGS
Doctoral Student
Department of Sociology
Case Western Reserve University
Cleveland, OH

Harry R. Moody, PhD
Senior Associate
International Longevity
   Center
Palisades, NY

**Nancy Morrow-Howell, MSW,
   PhD**
Ralph and Muriel Pumphery
   Professor of Social Work
George Warren Brown School
   of Social Work
Washington University
St. Louis, MO

Carol M. Musil, PhD, RN
Associate Professor
Frances Payne Bolton
   School of Nursing
Case Western Reserve
   University
Cleveland, OH

Silvia Orsulic-Jeras, MA
Myers Research Institute of
   the Menorah Park Center
   for Senior Living
Beachwood, OH

Grace J. Petot, MS
Assistant Professor Emerita
Department of Nutrition and
    Laboratory of Neurogeriatics
School of Medicine
Case Western Reserve University
Cleveland, OH

**Beverly L. Roberts, PhD, RN,
    FAAN, FGSA**
Arline H. & Curtis F. Garvin
    Professor and Administrative
    Associate to the Dean for
    Special Programs
Frances Payne Bolton School
    of Nursing
Case Western Reserve University
Cleveland, OH

Michael Sherraden, MSW, PhD
Benjamin E. Youngdahl
    Professor of Social
    Development
George Warren Brown
    School of Social Work
Washington University
St. Louis, MO

Eleanor P. Stoller, PhD
Selah Chamberlain Professor
    of Sociology
Associate Director
Center of Aging and Health
Case Western Reserve University
Cleveland, OH

Fengyan Tang, MSW
PhD Student
George Warren Brown School
    of Social Work
Washington University
St. Louis, MO

Camille B. Warner, PhD
Project Manager
Intergenerational Caregiving
    Study
Frances Payne Bolton School
    of Nursing
Case Western Reserve University
Cleveland, OH

Noah J. Webster, BA
Doctoral Student
Department of Sociology
Case Western Reserve University
Cleveland, OH

Catherine Whitehouse, PhD
Principal Teacher and Executive
    Director
The Intergenerational School
Cleveland, OH

Foreword

Aging is both a biological process and a sociological phenomenon. As a biological process, it can be seen as beginning at birth or conception and unfolding throughout the life span. In this way, biological changes affect the individual organism, leading to a variety of changes throughout life, from growth and maturation through the child-rearing years and into the period known as old-age or senescence.

Understanding these changes over time, and ameliorating those that are undesirable, is an important part of understanding aging research. Equally important is the need to understand the impact of the aging process on the individual within the context of society. What values and roles are assigned to the individual based upon chronological age? What expectations does society have for people? And are there resources available to help people meet these expectations?

As overall population aging takes place, such questions become more pressing. In the first decades of the 21st century, these are pressing questions indeed. Throughout the world—in the industrialized world and, increasingly, in poorer countries—we are seeing perhaps the greatest demographic shift ever. Life expectancies have exploded, both at birth and at older ages. People over the age of 100, once seen only rarely, have become much more common. Large percentages of the population are entering the period traditionally known as "aged," making the traditional age pyramid much more rectangular and changing the ratios among various population segments. The traditional three-generation family is becoming stretched into four and sometimes five generations. Although often presented as a "crisis," this demographic revolution is also one of the great successes of our time.

One of the challenges for society is deciding what this demographic change means and how we want to think about it. A quarter century ago, as the initial focus on the issue emerged, the clear focus was one of problems. Aging was seen as the cause of problems for society's elderly: high numbers living in poverty or with poor nutrition—inadequate availability of services to deal with long-term health care needs—lack of understanding of geriatric medicine and other special needs.

Although many of these issues still remain, there has been tremendous progress over the past quarter century on many fronts. We have learned a tremendous amount about many of the common diseases of aging. There have been significant policy victories, from improving the quality of long-term care facilities to improving recognition of and responses to elder abuse. Many people and institutions in our society can rightfully take pride in these accomplishments, from academicians to policy advocates.

As we have seen progress on this front, we have also seen additional developments that result from thinking about aging in a new way. Although seemingly diverse in approaches, these efforts share some similarities. For one, they include efforts to change negative stereotypes of aging and to highlight new models of aging. There is also a focus on better understanding of the interplay of aging as a process and disease—for example, to what degree does disease actually produce the changes attributed to the aging process? Similarly, how might alterations in social roles lead to new approaches to well-being among the aged?

Many foundations played a significant role in the progress we have made over the years by supporting research and training in geriatrics, by improvements in long-term and palliative care, by supporting public policy analysis work, and by promoting studies of significant ethical issues. Thus, foundations deserve some of the credit for the progress we have made in an aging society.

Increasingly, foundations are taking the lead in supporting the new and emerging view of aging, one that views aging as a tremendous societal opportunity. They are promoting efforts that can lead to a tremendous growth in opportunities for older persons to give back through volunteerism and engagement in community life. They encourage efforts to untangle the impact of disease from the normal aging process. Teaching people how to plan for their own retirement and discover new approaches to lifelong learning is another area of foundation support. Communities, as well, are being assisted in adjusting to the current aging boom, just as they adjusted to the baby boom in the mid-1950s.

Are there dangers in this new approach? Of course there are. We can forget that despite significant improvements, there are still too many people who are poor, alone, and hurting. If not cautious, we can allow the "successful aging" movement to turn into a celebration of the fittest or wealthiest, while those facing challenges are blamed for their own misfortunes. This can lead to "blaming the victim," in which people in poor health or with insufficient resources are said to have caused their situation and to be undeserving of assistance. These are real concerns, ones that we forget at our own peril.

On the other hand, the concepts of successful aging, when applied appropriately, can be powerful levers for change. They allow people to recognize that biological aging is only one influence on their future, and that people also have opportunities to shape their futures as they go forward. The contemporary concepts of aging help society to recognize that people are likely to have a long period of relatively good health. Longevity provides the opportunity for elders to take the roads not traveled when younger and to make long-deferred commitments to education or service. The concept of successful aging encourages us to see society not merely as the problem solver, but also as providing the support to allow people to anticipate and plan for their own aging. Finally, positive aging concepts show the interactions among broader societal decisions about roles and opportunities as well as the biological aging process itself.

We are on a road that no society has taken before. The challenges of an aging society lie before us. Increasingly, we are seeing the opportunities of an aging society as well. The better we understand the interplay of aging challenges and supportive services, the better prepared we will be for the road that lies before us, both as a society and as individuals within it.

ROBERT E. ECKARDT, DrPH
Vice President for Programs and Evaluation
The Cleveland Foundation

Acknowledgments

This edited volume results from a 1-day-conference, "Successful Aging Through the Life Span—Intergenerational Issues in Health," which was held on October 7, 2002, in Cleveland, Ohio. The editors wish to thank members of the planning committee for their invaluable assistance in the development of the program. Thanks also to—among others—the A.M. McGregor Home, Cleveland, Ohio; Janssen Pharmaceutica Products, Pfizer Inc.; the Mt. Sinai Health Care Foundation, Cleveland, Ohio; and St. Luke's Foundation of Cleveland, Ohio—for their generous support for the conference.

Our special thanks to Sandra Hanson, the University Center on Aging and Health's department assistant, for executing the myriad tasks involved in bringing the conference to fruition and for compiling and editing this manuscript; and to Diane Ferris, manager of the University Center on Aging and Health. We are also appreciative of Charles L. Onyett, a student assistant, for his help with section introductions.

MAY L. WYKLE, PHD, RN, FAAN, FGSA
PETER J. WHITEHOUSE, MD, PHD
DIANA L. MORRIS, PHD, RN, FAAN

Introduction

The Frances Payne Bolton School of Nursing and the University Center on Aging and Health at Case Western Reserve University sponsored the 14th Florence Cellar Gerontology Conference on October 7, 2002, in Cleveland, Ohio. The conference aimed to bring scholars and practitioners from the community together to examine ideas of successful aging and productive intergenerational relationships. To reach a wider audience and disseminate the thinking and research that is being done for successful aging and intergenerational health, the issues and ideas that were discussed at the conference are presented in this book. A greater awareness of the gerontological issues will lead to more in-depth research, better outcomes, and more widespread knowledge of the problems and solutions associated with aging.

Exploring concepts and practices of successful and productive aging, identifying the best practices to enhance successful aging, examining trends in intergenerational caregiving, and defining the roles and responsibilities across the stages of life are some of the issues that were confronted at the conference. Sessions were held to discuss factors that contribute to successful aging, dealing specifically with exercise and nutrition, as well as with established stereotypes of aging. Other sessions concentrated on specific intergenerational issues, such as the role of children and adults in interaction with elders as well as the role of care services in helping elders to remain active and stay involved in the social realm.

The conference reflected the vision of Florence Cellar, a nurse who wished to improve the quality of life for older persons, and both academic and community leaders actively engaged in discussions on successful aging. The purpose of this book is to present the major foci of the conference—namely, the following:

- To explore concepts and practices of successful and productive aging
- To identify best practices to enhance successful aging
- To examine trends in intergenerational caregiving
- To define the roles and responsibilities across the life span
- To exercise imagination about intergenerational health promotion
- To describe the diversity of paths to successful aging

PART I

Health and Productivity— Challenging the Mystique of Longevity

May L. Wykle

This first section deals primarily with the idea of the "new gerontology": the interpretation of aging as a positive, productive process that moves away from the notion of the aging process as a slow and steady decline in health and productivity. The following chapters focus on two main ideas: how to promote and enrich the health of the elderly population, and how to better utilize them as productive members of society. In examining these issues, this section confronts problems such as culturally entrenched prejudices against the idea of incorporating the elders into the workforce, and the resistance of society to recognizing that aging is not an automatic winding down in life but a chance to be just as active, if not more so, than in previous life stages.

In the first chapter, Juengst describes the argument within the gerontological community for breaking down the stigma associated with aging and replacing it with a more positive outlook. This issue is approached from two different angles: first examining the arguments of those attempting to distinguish aging from disease, and second, using fictional examples to imagine a world where these arguments might be true. Juengst analyzes the perspectives of clinicians and social scientists on aging, which are mostly dependent on life experience versus the perspectives of basic scientists, who focus more on wide-ranging biological trends. Emphasized throughout is the distinction between aging and senescence; the former is defined as the number of years lived, the latter as the highly relative physical and biological changes the body undergoes while aging. Ultimately, Juengst argues that none of the theory and research proves wholly satisfactory and that gerontology has the challenge of explaining how aging can be a healthy process without disregarding senescence. He cautions against jumping too quickly at conclusions about aging changes.

A different aspect of aging is taken up in the second chapter by Morrow-Howell, Tang, Kim, Lee, and Sherraden on how to promote successful aging. The authors claim that activity during life is strongly tied to longer and healthier life spans. For those in more advanced stages of life, the authors focus on those activities in which these elders are most commonly engaged, termed "productive activities." These activities include volunteering, working, and caregiving, all socially beneficial activities that are not beyond the scope of the individual. The chapter provides an in-depth statistical analysis of the levels of individual social involvement, awareness, and action. The analysis uncovers a need for better development of programs and support for the elders to facilitate their involvement in activities that are both beneficial to them and to society. Such facilitation by society would result in the realization of a "third age" in the human life cycle.

Moody, in the third chapter, takes a more philosophical approach to the aging process, claiming that the mindset of the older person can improve one's state of health. Going against the widely held notion that aging is a negative process, Moody distinguishes two kinds of aging: "successful aging" and "productive aging." Successful aging is sustained health later in life, while productive aging is a continued commitment to society through volunteerism and other forms of contribution. Moody goes on to examine how successful aging can be enriched by examining two philosophical outlooks: (1) holding on to values from middle age through the later stages of life, and (2) "decrement with compensation," which involves adapting to the changes of aging. Citing various examples from persons such as Beethoven and Picasso, Moody's argument moves toward the decrement-with-compensation outlook as being more successful and less static than merely aging successfully that allows elders to maintain a positive yet flexible outlook in the face of obstacles. Thus, a flexible, positive attitude is the key to successful aging.

CHAPTER 1

Can Aging Be Interpreted as a Healthy, Positive Process?

Eric T. Juengst

Ever since the MacArthur Foundation's catalytic collection of research projects on "successful aging" in the 1980s, there has been an effort within gerontology to destigmatize aging and reinterpret it as a normal, healthy, and even positive feature of the human life cycle (Rowe & Kahn, 1997; Gergen & Gergen, 2001). The chapters in this volume represent the cutting edge of that movement (see Moody, e.g.). For these gerontologists, the aging process, far from being pathological, deserves as much cultural celebration as we give to the complementary processes of growth and maturation. For them, the fact that normal aging has become medicalized and pathologized is only an unfortunate artifact of a cultural bias in favor of youth and is a particularly stigmatizing feature of the ageism that infects our society (Hazan, 1994).

Gerontology's efforts to put a positive face on aging are philosophically interesting because, as others have pointed out, human aging looks very pathological from most theoretical perspectives (Caplan, 1982). From the perspective of the biomedical model of pathology, human senescence carries all the hallmarks of a disease process: specific underlying molecular changes create abnormalities in cells that inhibit the functional efficiency and structural resiliency of tissues and organs, causing disabilities, deformities, and distress at the systemic level that fall into stable patterns of specific signs, symptoms, and complaints (Thagard, 1999). From clinical medicine's perspective, aging does produce the cardinal indications for health care interventions: pain, fatigue, sensory loss, and functional decline (Cassell, 1982). Sociologically speaking, aging warrants social roles that relieve one of normal work responsibilities, and it invokes caregiving duties amongst one's friends and families, just as sickness does (Shenk and Achenbaum, 1994). Culturally, both aging and disease are understood in our society primarily through their association with death: illness symbolizes for us our vulnerability, and aging is emblematic of the inevitability of our demise (Cole & Gadow, 1986). Even the so-called virtues of aging—the equanimity, wisdom, and generativity that can come with aging—are products of the same kind of character-building that is ascribed to disease: they are virtues purported to flow from suffering and learning to live within limits (Kass, 2002). Admittedly, these perspectives may be influenced by the same antiaging bias that the proponents of successful aging would like to expose and refute. But they still pose a formidable phalanx of challenges to their effort.

Is it really possible to consistently and coherently reinterpret aging in a way that does not tie the process to the endpoint of death, that does not impose the sick role on the elderly, and that can interpret the biological changes of the aging process in "demedicalized" value—neutral or positive terms? In this essay, I explore this question in two different ways. In the first section below, I look at the arguments of those who seek to distinguish aging from disease to test them for their intellectual soundness. In the second section, I try to envision the realization of their dream, through imaginative fiction. Can one imagine a society in which senescence is regarded as a positive human developmental process in the same way we regard human growth and maturation? In the final section, I draw from both exercises to express my doubts. Although there are many ways in which the experience of aging could be improved, I think in the end it is very difficult to interpret human aging as a process we should admire, facilitate, and sustain.

TWO APPROACHES TO NORMALIZING AGING

The attempt to reinterpret human aging as a healthy, positive process takes place at two levels in the literature: There are arguments advanced by clinicians and social scientists framed in terms of the lived experience of older people and arguments advanced by basic scientists framed in terms of the biological phenomena involved in human aging.

For the clinicians and social scientists, one major conceptual move has been to distinguish between the concepts of aging and of senescence. As the proponents of successful aging put it, in scientific terms, one's age is a measure of the number of years one has lived. Since aging occurs as a function of additional years since birth, strictly speaking, everyone ages at the same rate. Senescence, on the other hand, refers to the biological and physiological changes that occur in an individual as he or she ages. Senescence is highly variable, and proceeds at different rates in different people. (Rowe & Kahn, 1997, p. 208.)

This distinction suggests to the proponents of successful aging the theoretical possibility of aging without senescence—or at least without the "usual" senescent processes that give aging its association with pathology. They say:

> usual aging involves two key sets of problems. First, many body organs—including the kidneys, heart, and lungs—gradually lose strength with advancing age. Immune function also declines with age. These changes place the elderly at risk for disease or dysfunction, especially in the presence of major stress. The second set of problems that develop in usual aging relate to the buildup of many risky characteristics such as high levels of blood fats and sugar, hypertension and so on. . . . Just as no two people are alike, so their physiological health—that is, the functional capacity of their major body organs—varies dramatically. This variability between individuals tends to increase with advancing age. (Rowe & Kahn, 1997, pp. 54–57)

Since Rowe and Kahn believe that "risk factors that comprise the 'usual aging' syndrome are modifiable," (p. 57), this allows them to propose a new ideal of successful aging for gerontological research and practice: the addition of years to life without concomitant pathological senescence: "We therefore define successful aging as the ability to maintain three key behaviors or characteristics: low risk of disease and disease-related disability; high mental and physical function; and active engagement in life" (Rowe & Kahn, 1997, p. 38).

Of course, adopting a strictly chronological definition of aging, so that even Peter Pan could be said to be successfully aging as he adds years to his eternal youth, sidesteps the real issue. In defending the normality of human aging, the challenge is precisely to explain senescence—the biological changes that come with human duration through time—in a nonpathological way. Presumably, since Rowe and Kahn disparage gerontologists that proceed "as if successful aging were merely aging as little as possible" (p. 52), these authors must hold that there are senescent biological changes that are not part of the (pathological) "usual aging syndrome" and would be compatible with the preservation of the traits that constitute successful aging. But they do not discuss these, and it is not clear what those positive senescent changes might be or how they contribute to successful aging—that is, to lowering the risk of disability and disease, improving mental and physical functioning, and enhancing active engagement with life.

The psychologists Mary Gergen and Kenneth Gergen take the experiential approach further in developing their vision of "positive aging". They argue that the account of senescence that emphasizes decline, degeneration, and decrepitude is a socially negotiated fiction produced by the individualist tradition in American culture and the Protestant work ethic." In fact, they assert that "there is no process of aging in itself; the discourse of aging is born of interpersonal relationships within a given culture at a given time" (Gergen & Gergen, 2001, p. 6).

Against this backdrop, they accuse existing gerontological research of thoroughgoing ascertainment bias: "That is, of the many complexes of dimensions of aging, researchers select out only those that demonstrate decline. Why, one wonders, is not more attention paid to forms of enhancement?" (Gergen & Gergen, p. 8). To suggest the kinds of enhancements that aging might provide, the authors sketch a "lifespan diamond" of four mutually reinforcing factors shown to improve human quality of life: "physical well being, positive mental status, engaging activity, and relational resources" (p. 10). The "critical fulcrum" of this system is a person's relational resources, and this set of resources ("supportive family and friends, conversational partners, mediated companions"), they say, has the potential to keep increasing with age, to the point that any declines in physical well being are completely offset and both mental status and social engagement ultimately enhanced. In support of this claim, the Gergens turn to the recent research within positive psychology that links longevity and health to altruism, social involvement, and interpersonal generativity. Aging, then, can be reinterpreted as essentially a process of accumulating and cultivating relationships, in which, when it goes well, the experience of physical decline is eclipsed by the happiness and stimulation of human interaction.

This is an appealing vision of the ingredients of human flourishing and resonates well with much of contemporary philosophical thought about the role of positive interpersonal relationships in human affairs (Post, 2003). However, exactly the same case could be made to promote the accumulation of wealth as the true point of aging. Wealth can also increase indefinitely through time, and it also allows one to offset any physical declines by enhancing the other facets of the life diamond—including one's relational resources. Power and knowledge also share these virtues. However, it is not terribly appealing to have to say that what is good about aging is that it allows one time to accumulate power, wealth, and knowledge so that enough relational resources can be acquired to offset any physical declines that might also occur during one's lifetime. By identifying the factors that make it possible to flourish in spite of senescence, these gerontologists have tacitly admitted that senescence itself is not a form of human flourishing. Once again, the only way this approach allows aging to escape that stigma is to deny that senescence and aging are essentially linked.

Basic scientists who study the biology of aging take another approach to this problem. First, they acknowledge senescence as the essential aspect of the phenomenon they seek to explain. Moreover, they are forthright in describing senescence with words that convey loss, decline, damage, and vulnerability. Thus, for example, one consensus statement of biogerontologists reports that "We think of aging as the accumulation of random damage in the building blocks of life—especially to DNA, certain proteins, carbohydrates and lipids—that begins early in life and eventually exceeds the bodies' self-repair capabilities" (Olshanksy, Hayflick, & Carnes, 2002). Biogerontologist Leonard Hayflick is even more succinct. He defines aging as "the normal biological processes that are collectively the single greatest risk factor for the pathologies of old age" (Hayflick, 2001). Nevertheless, these scientists think that it is a mistake to conceptualize these processes themselves as health problems, because they are ubiquitous phenomena that have an ecological role to play at levels of biological organization above the individual. For example, what distinguishes aging from disease for Hayflick is simply its universality. Hayflick writes:

> Aging is not a disease because, unlike any disease, age changes have the following characteristics: (1) they occur in every animal that reaches a fixed size in adulthood, (2) they cross virtually every species barrier; (3) they occur only after sexual maturation, (4) they occur in animals

removed from the wild and protected by humans even when that species has not been known to have experienced aging during any of its previous thousands or millions of years of existence, (5) they increase vulnerability to death in 100 percent of the animals in which the changes occur, and (6) they occur in both animate and inanimate objects (Hayflick, 2001, p. 22).

There are several ideas at play in this argument. By including the deterioration of inanimate objects under his definition of aging, Hayflick expands the term to mean the universal increase of entropy required by the second law of thermodynamics: an expansion that not only demedicalizes but also debiologizes aging in a way that gives it no particular role in the human life story. Aging is not a disease because it is not even a biological process: it is simply a token of the universal decay that sets in once the evolutionarily protected energies of sexual maturation stop holding it at bay in adult animals.

But even if entropic decay is universal and inevitable amongst adult animals, it can still be harmful. All adult animals (and inanimate objects) will also undergo the molecular changes associated with freezing when subjected to subfreezing temperatures, also with 100% risk of death, but hypothermia is not considered healthy as a consequence. If nature can find ways to swim upstream against entropy for the first dozen years of human life, why shouldn't we attempt to extend the swim thereafter, just as we take steps to avoid hypothermia?

Moreover, if it is only the universality of senescence that secures its normality for humans, what happens to that status as we acquire the ability to make it optional? At any given time there are, of course, millions of animals who grow to a fixed size that have not yet begun to show the signs of aging, despite the second law of thermodynamics: the prepubescent young. Once biological senescence, as we have known it, is no longer inevitable, that generation need make a virtue of necessity no longer.

It is at this point that others will marshal evolutionary hypotheses to argue that, whether or not aging is good for the individual, it serves a crucial role in the health of human populations by providing a caste of postreproductive dependent domestic caregivers and, ultimately, by keeping populations below the carrying capacity of the biosphere (Kirkwood, 1999). This may be true, of course, but the same population benefits can also be provided by interpersonal violence, slavery, epidemic disease, and starvation. Even if these phenomena contribute, in the long run, to the survival of the species and the health of the biosphere, they are usually listed amongst the human experiences we would like to avoid, if at all possible, both for ourselves and for others. If we have to stretch this far from ordinary morality in order to see the bright side of aging, it is likely that most would forego the exercise.

In summation, neither the successful aging paradigm nor the biogerontologists' "universal aging" approach is entirely satisfying in reforming our tendency to think about human aging as a pathological process worthy of medical intervention. Is it really possible to offer a positive account of aging that could render senescence as culturally attractive as maturation—that is, to hold out the possibility that growing old might be valued as much as growing up is as a stage of human biological development? The psychologists, Gergen and Gergen, endorse the use of "appreciative inquiry" techniques to help people reinterpret aging, explaining that "the challenge is for them to tell stories in which people locate in such events [wrinkled faces and sagging bodies, chronic disease, disability, and the death of intimate others] opportunities for significant development, creativity, invigoration or inspiration" (p. 15). In the next section, I follow their advice and attempt to tell just such a story.

BUTTERFLIES ASCENDANT

"There goes that Vanessa! I swear she gains another year every month!"

"Yes, well, she's certainly well ripened for her age. You know that gorgeous silver comes right out of a bottle."

Edith turned back from the antique store window to take another look at the owl she had been holding up to the light. It was a 19th century bronze Owl of Minerva. The patina glowed like polished wood, and it had the comforting heft of something stable and enduring. Edith collected owl images, and this one would be the best yet, if only she could afford it. She sighed and set it carefully back down on the barrister bookcase, where it had been brooding over a family of brass candlesticks, souvenir pyramids, and pocket watches.

"I know just how you feel," she thought. "How can we fly with the owls with these families hemming us in?" She glanced down at her daughter at her feet, who was beginning to whine for attention again. She had already left viscous little fingerprints all over the glass front of the bookcase, and now she obviously thought she was too far from her walker to get back by herself. When she raised her bubbly, stubby hands up to Edith, her sour smell came with them.

******

Graceful folds of soft skin invited his fingers to trace their lines. An autumnal landscape of freckles and moles faded to snowy cream in the places ordinarily covered by clothes. Her eyes were deep and smiling, set in traceries of laugh lines that conveyed their invitation to every corner of her face. Her hair was cropped to a fog-gray carpet on the facing side of her head; on the other, it fell in a fluid steel drape across her far shoulder. It was one of the most provocative images Gerry had ever seen on a bus-stop billboard, and he couldn't keep his eyes off it. On the one hand, it was shocking, bordering on soft-core gero-porn. It was shameless the way advertisers pandered to society's obsession with age. This model was old enough to be his mother. On the other hand, he had to admit it stirred him.

He wasn't a hardened gerophile, but there was something in the persistent sexuality of the image that reminded him of Nabokov's LoGranda. Why is it men are excited by women who are sexually inviting after their reproductive years? Certainly, the Internet is full of Web sites devoted to naked middle-aged women made up to look older than they are, carrying garden trowels or memoirs or other normal tools of old age.

Still, whatever sordid psychological buttons the billboard pushed, one had to admit that the model was flawless. There were probably rich young women right now showing her photo to their cosmetic surgeons, seeking to replicate the intricate calligraphy of her face. Gerry saw the bus turn the corner and stood up with a shiver of relief.

******

Bob originally went into higher education because he liked being around the seniors on the university campus. Their insights and ideas, crystallized and anchored by their experience, were a constant food for thought, and their general disregard for the conventions of their juniors was refreshing. How ironic, then, to end up stuck in a community college, essentially providing day care for a bunch of twig-in-the-wind adolescents with nothing better to do.

Today, he was going to try a topic that would be a sure-fire discussion catalyst amongst mature students: the growing debate over the relative allocation of scare medical resources to those in the first year of life. Bioethicists were pointing out that while high-tech medical institutions poured an ever-larger share of the health care dollar into salvaging frail newborns, funding for basic preventive eldercare was going lacking in many communities. A baby, of course, is a renewable resource; when any elder's unique lifelong accumulation of experience, relationships, and memories is extinguished, however, it is gone forever. Pointing to Nature's age-old wisdom of "throwing back" infants too premature or defective to flourish in old age, these authors argue that society should set limits on biomedicine's infatuation with life-for-life's sake and the technologies that emerge from it.

To this, Bob thought, his students would probably grunt and stare blankly. After all, they have yet to even experience child-bearing, and the inevitable pain of deciding to place a baby in a home or have it put down, much less the fine-grained joys of maturity. Caught in the grip of their consumerism and petty gossip, their minds are, as someone once said, "indistinguishable blurs upon which nothing imprints, driven before a hormonal wind."

******

Edith had to admit that, as much as she loved her, her daughter was disgusting. Janet's fixed smile seemed to agree. But it wasn't the baby's sticky skin or swollen face that bothered her as much as her attitude: that self-centered cranky neediness. She knew her daughter couldn't help it yet, but it was so rude and so embarrassing to have to do personal caregiving in public like this.

Still, family ties were strong for Edith. She was not the sort of mother who could just park her children in a nursery, as Janet had. Even though the extra caregiving took time from playing with her own mom, she felt an anticipatory gratitude obliging her to see to her child's rearing personally. Someday, after all, the baby's life would revolve around Edith.

"Are you crones ready yet?" Janet and Edith's mothers sailed out of the back room. They were beaming at the small generosity of extending maturity to their middle-aged daughters. "We've pretty much exhausted this place."

Edith laughed. It was flattering to be treated like one of the crones by her mother, even though she was over 60 years away from the century mark. It would still be a while before she would lose her rubbery, tight skin and could get away with flouncing around without her maturizing undergarments like her elders. She touched the penciled lines on her cheek and offered another silent plea to Grandmother Mary that she inherit her mother's great natural wrinkles. At just 25 years away, her mom was at the peak of her adult beauty. From here on, she would get cuter and cuter, in the wizened, enthralling way of old people, but at the moment, she was in her glory. Well, she deserved it.

"Mom, what do you think of this owl?"

******

Bob spotted the new owl about halfway through dinner.

"Whoa!" He sat back in his chair. "Where did that come from?"

"Mom and I found it today at that antique place on Main. Isn't it perfect?"

"And did your mom pay for it as well? Come on, Edie, you know we are barely making it as it is. How much was it?"

"Actually, Mom did buy it for me, out of her own money. It was a gift, for heaven's sake!"

"Well, I'm sorry to snap, then. I guess I'm still a cranky teenager after all. It's just that we are only just beginning to get out of the hole, and I feel responsible."

"Honey, you know you don't have to apologize for coming out of pretirement so late: you might never have gotten out if you hadn't gone to graduate school. I don't really see you as a slow-food store clerk or a nursery aide."

"But I am a nursery aide! You should have seen me pulling baby teeth today trying to get a discussion going in my class. I was giving them Caplan's arguments that we should really admit that growth is pathological, and even though it was basically about them, they couldn't have been more apathetic."

"You philosophers! How could growth be a disease? Everything grows."

"Exactly! And growth is the death of everything; you can only buck the second law of thermodynamics for so long before you pay the price. In nature, unbridled growth inevitably leads to ecological collapse. In people, that collapse is disease. Think about it. What is cancer? Uncontrolled growth. What is infection? Unrestrained growth. What is mental illness? The malignant growth of obsessions, depressions, regressions, and fears. Why are the diseases of childhood so virulent and acute, compared to the chronic diseases of maturity? Because they are functions of immaturity: cell division gone haywire, immune systems stretched too thin, suicidal ideation unbuffered by experience and relationships. Granted, we tend to treat individual growth-associated health problems as if they were independent, but in terms of health-risk factors alone, it's a relief to stop growing and start aging."

"Honey, you are lecturing again. Slow down and eat your dinner."

******

Gerry got back into the lab early the next day. The problem was a tough lump to squeeze, but he was finally starting to see some diamond sparkle in the coal. He worked to compress the morbidities of growth back as far as possible into youth, without creating other health problems in the process. He had a nice progeric mouse strain now, the pups of which began to show the healthy signs of aging—slowed metabolism, reduced cell division, more careful movement—as soon as they were weaned. His technique for peeling the telomeres in the stem cells that became their progenitor seemed to work. However, the animal's growth remained, if anything, a more precipitous process, leading to significantly more stillbirths and congenital defects.

If only there were a way to decelerate the gestational process so that development could move more sedately, he might be able to achieve the Holy Grail of developmental biology, which says that healthy animals are sexually mature at birth and begin aging immediately thereafter, even as they continue to grow to adult sizes. Admittedly, to translate this into a practical early-aging intervention for human beings would require still further steps. The main thing would be to postpone the neonates' fertility and sexuality until they had matured enough. On the bright side, there would be no reason to stick to nature's barbaric time line on that score. Rather than torture adolescents with these traits, they could be postponed as far into adulthood as the aging process would permit.

Gerry leaned back in his chair and smiled to himself. What would philosopher Bob think about that, if he knew what was coming down the pike?! There were still those who thought that the aches, pains and deadly eruptions of growth were something that should be tolerated just because they were "natural" and "instructive." But he had yet to find an adolescent who would not happily forego the "wisdom" acquired by losing control of one's mind and body if the opportunity to start aging gracefully presented itself ahead of schedule. There were plenty of normal aging pains to be endured to cultivate the epic virtues of empathy and equanimity, and, Lord knows, still enough passion and heartbreak to inspire the sleepiest poet.

This reminded him of Vanessa. Vanessa, whose name means "butterfly." The butterfly, nature's swooping shouts in praise of life's grand finale, the very symbol of successful aging. If only he could catch her.

CONCLUSION

Edith's world is as close to a mirror image of our own as I could make it, and, obviously, some features of it are not very realistic. But even this relatively strained attempt to envision a world in which aging is socially reconstructed as positive is thought provoking. It illustrates the Gergens' point that there is no single truth about aging, but, rather, "an array of possible worlds from which people can draw as their lives unfold"(Gergen & Gergen, 2001, p. 20). Their example of this point could be discussing Gerry's reaction to the billboard model:

Is wrinkled skin necessarily a deficit, an alienating and distancing feature of the face? In fact, many people find wrinkled skin quite beautiful, a signal of a life well lived, wisdom, and special insight. Whether a body is beautiful or desirable is not inherent in the body itself but in the domain of relations that define the body in this way or that. It is in this way that the residents of many retirement communities are successful in shedding the common cultural definitions of beauty and desirability (Gergen & Gergen, 2001, p. 13).

On the other hand, Edith's world is clearly not a utopia, and it immediately highlights two important concerns about the ultimate implications of the "positive aging" movement in gerontology.

The first complaint about the society I have imagined is that its members admire the aging process at the expense of youth and growth, simply mirroring in reverse the prejudices of our own society. Is that necessary, either psychologically or logically? It is true that one cannot value something without proportionally disvaluing its opposite: valuation implies a "lexical ordering" of goods, which in turn implies a relative ranking of our preferences.

Psychologically, we do often polarize such value rankings, so that what is not ideal comes to be perceived, irrationally, as distinctly negative. To that extent, we should perhaps expect a "pro-aging" society to develop a corresponding disvaluing of youth and growth. However, perhaps senescence and growth are not the only possible poles to contrast in a social assessment of aging. For example, one logically coherent alternative would be a society that admired all kinds of human change over time and disvalued developmental stasis or stagnation. The cultural tenacity of Cartesian dualism often inclines us to think of aging as a bodily process that compromises and eventually eclipses a transcendent, personal self that, even if it evolves to maturity, remains stable throughout adulthood. If, instead, we lived in a society in which we took the observation that "he's not the same person he once was" as good news rather than an expression of concern, we might have room for a system that could equally value both growth and senescence.

The second question raised by my thought experiment concerns the status of death in a society like the one I've imagined. Would they accept and celebrate death in old age as the telos of the aging process, as we celebrate a birth as the genesis of a new life? Or would they lament death as the tragic interruption of the aging process, like we regret the death of the young? Without a religious vision of what comes after death, the former risks generating a macabre and ultimately depressing worldview, not unlike that of some 20th century existentialists. If it is the latter, however, another unattractive prospect suggests itself—that a society that actually idealized aging would invest heavily in attempts to prolong the process of senescence as long as possible in the face of death.

As Bob's mouse experiments suggest, the goal of biogerontological research in this society would be to extend, not compress, senescence, so that people could enjoy the enhancing, positive changes of extreme old age earlier and longer. The outcome, of course, would be many more frail, dependent, and compromised elderly rather than an increase in the vigorous, semisenesced exemplars of successful aging. But for a consistent and robust pro-aging value system, that would be the right outcome, and the social costs of such a system are merely the price of being true to the belief that aging is a positive, normal, healthy human phenomenon.

In the end, this analysis leaves me doubtful that a positive vision of aging ultimately makes sense. So far, as I have tried to show above, the formal attempts of gerontologists and biogerontologists to reinterpret human aging as a positive phenomenon have not been entirely successful. Senescence may be a perfectly natural, universal, inevitable, highly variable, character-building process, but it remains a series of functional losses that eventually prove fatal for everyone who experiences them. As religious traditions around the world demonstrate, it is possible to build a social system of beliefs and relationships that can compensate for those losses and reframe death as a transition rather than as an endpoint. But as long as the goal of medicine is to reduce the risk of functional losses and death, the aging process will continue to be a conceptually coherent and strategic target for medical intervention—in short, as legitimate a health problem as smoking, alcoholism, or unsafe sexual practices.

Moreover, if the new gerontology were successful beyond its wildest dreams in reconstructing society's vision of aging, that success would be accompanied by some vexing new philosophical problems. Can we raise up the aging process without simultaneously devaluing youth, growth, and development? Growth and senescence are both teleological concepts in our culture, but with very different end-points: maturity and death. If we call the entire human life course "growth," what does it grow toward? Without an accompanying spiritual vision that can suggest a transcendent afterlife, positive aging risks promoting an incomplete narrative for human life, in which the flourishing we associate with maturity is simply replaced by the finality of death.

Indeed, as Edith's world suggests, a society that treasures aging would probably find death in old age even more offensive than our youth culture does and would devote its efforts to prolonging the process of senescence as much as possible. But even given a society that enjoyed the social resources to insure that the elderly themselves do not experience their declines negatively, the prospect of what has been called the "national nursing home scenario" (Fukyama, 2002) seems distinctly at odds with the original intentions of those who promote the new gerontology."

There is no doubt that we could be more balanced in our cultural assessment of aging than we are, and the notions of successful and of positive aging offer useful rallying points for improving the experience of aging in our society. It does appear, however, that the proponents of the new gerontology need to take care to develop their conceptual claims further, with two major challenges in mind. The first challenge is to show how we can understand the aging process as a healthy process without jettisoning biological senescence as a major part of the phenomena to be explained. So far, neither the social scientific nor the biological defenses of the normality of aging have succeeded in demonstrating how senescence could be health promoting for those experiencing it. The second challenge is to think about the downstream implications of the reconstruction of aging for other features of our value system. Like any revolution, there is always the danger of getting what one wishes for and then finding the new regime even more oppressive than the old.

ACKNOWLEDGMENTS

This essay is the hybrid offspring of a discussion session at the Successful Aging Conference that inspired this book and a writing exercise undertaken at an National Institute of Health (NIH) Summer Seminar sponsored by the Hiram College Center for Literature and Medicine. My efforts to combine these reflections were underwritten by a research grant from the National Institute of Aging and the National Human Genome Research Institute (R01-AG20916-01). I am indebted to my coinvestigators in that research, to my colleagues at Hiram, to the Successful Aging Conference organizers, and to Peter Whitehouse, as one of all of the above and as editor, for encouraging this intellectual crossbreeding experiment.

REFERENCES

Caplan, A..(1982). The unnaturalness of aging: A sickness unto death? In A. Caplan, H. T. Engelhardt, & J. McCartney (Eds.), *Concepts of health and disease: Interdisciplinary perspectives* (pp. 331–345). Boston: Addison-Wesley.

Cassell, E., (1982). The nature of suffering and the goals of medicine. *New England Journal of Medicine, 306,* 639–645.

Cole, T., & Gadow, S. (Eds.). (1986). *What does it mean to grow old? Reflections from the humanities.* Durham, NC: Duke University Press.

Fukuyama, F. (2002). *Our posthuman future: Consequences of the biotechnology revolution.* New York: Profile Books.

Gergen, M., & Gergen, K. (2001). Positive aging: New images for a new age. *Ageing International, 27,* 3–23.

Hayflick, L. (2001). Anti-aging medicine: Hype, hope and reality. *Generations, 24*(4), 20–27.

Hazan, H. (1994). *Old age: Constructions and deconstructions.* Cambridge, England: Cambridge University Press.

Kass, L. (2002). *Life, liberty and the defense of dignity: The challenge for bioethics.* San Francisco: Encounter Books.

Kirkwood, T. (1999). *Time of our lives: The science of human aging*. New York: Oxford University Press.

Olshansky, S. J., Hayflick, L., & Carnes, B. (2002). Position statement of human aging. *Journal of Gerontology: Biological Sciences, 57A*(8), B292–B297.

Post, S. (2003). *Unlimited love: Altruism, compassion, and service*. Philadelphia: Templeton Foundation Press.

Rowe, J., & Kahn, R. (1997). *Successful aging*. New York: Pantheon Books.

Shenk, D., & Achenbaum, W. A., (Eds.). (1994). *Changing perceptions of aging and the aged*. New York: Springer Publishing Co.

Thagard, P. (1999). *How scientists explain disease*. Princeton, NJ: Princeton University Press.

CHAPTER 2

Maximizing the Productive Engagement of Older Adults

Nancy Morrow-Howell, Fengyan Tang, Jeounghee Kim, MiJin Lee, and Michael Sherraden

A s discussed throughout this book, life expectancy has changed dramatically since the turn of the last century. According to the Center for Disease Control (1999), a person retiring at age 65 has another 18 years of life ahead. In the face of this longevity, gerontology scholars have focused on well-being within those extended years. Data from the MacArthur Foundation Study of Successful Aging suggest that successful aging has three components: low probability of disease, high functioning, and active engagement with life (Rowe & Kahn, 1998). Further, Rowe and Kahn suggest that active engagement with life has two major components: activity and social support. Indeed, activity has long been associated with positive outcomes in later life (as cited in Everard, Lach, Fisher, & Baum, 2000). However, there are numerous types of activity. In fact, the "busy" ethic that has shaped modern retirement seems to suggest that any activity will do (Ekerdt, 1986). But Freedman (2001) argues that all activity is not created equal—to the individual, to the family, or to society.

This chapter focuses on a certain subset of activities—namely, productive activity. There are many definitions of productive activity offered in the literature. We use a narrow definition offered by Bass, Caro, and Chen (1993): Productive activity is any activity that produces goods or services, whether paid for or not. Activities included in this definition are volunteering, working, and caregiving. These activities are clearly a subset of activities in which older adults engage, and they have a common element: social benefits and impacts that extend beyond the individual.

Older adults engaged in these productive activities are performing valued functions to society. In fact, it is argued that there will be increased demand for elders in these roles in future years. The labor market will demand longer work lives (Mor-Barak & Wilson, in press). Growing social problems and reduced public expenditures will demand increased volunteerism (Abraham, Arrington, & Wasserbauer, 1996; Freedman, 1999). Increased numbers of the oldest old will require a larger force of caregivers. Thus, our society may require the productive engagement of older adults. Butler (1997) argues that we should transform retirement and extend work life and expand volunteer roles, for the benefit to the older adult as well as to society.

The purpose of this chapter is to overview current knowledge about productive engagement of older adults. We review three productive activities: working, volunteering, and caregiving. For each of these activities, we will review current levels of involvement of older Americans, policies that affect their involvement, and the effects of engagement on their well-being. We conclude with ideas about maximizing potential through increasing and improving the institutional capacity of our society to engage older adults in productive roles.

EMPLOYMENT

Current Levels of Engagement

During the past five decades, the labor participation rate of men has dramatically declined for both the 55- to 64-year-old age group and the 65 years and older group. At the same time, the participation rate of women aged 55 to 64 has almost doubled, and the rate for women over 65 has been relatively stable (Purcell, 2000).[1] In more recent years, the labor market participation rates of older adults have been steady, indicating that the long-term downward trend has finally leveled off. In fact, the most recent trend is that the employment rate of older adults, overall, is moving upward. Between 1999 and 2000, among the people 65 years old and older, both men and women increased their employment rates to 17.5 and 9.4, respectively. Notably, men in their 70s had a participation rate of more than 12% in 2000 (Purcell, 2000). In 2001, according to the Bureau of Labor Statistics (2003), 4.3 million (13.1%) Americans age 65 and over were in the labor force, constituting 3.0% of the U.S. labor force.

By and large, older adults' engagement in the labor market gradually decreases as age increases. While the proportion of full-time workers diminishes with age, that of part-time workers increases (Purcell, 2000; Hill, 2002). Older workers occupy a wide range of occupations. Approximately 62% of workers age 55 to 64 and 64 to 74 are employed in white-collar occupations, about 15% of workers between the age 65 and 74 are employed in service occupations, and nearly 23% of workers age 65 to 74 are engaged in blue-collar work (U.S. General Accounting Office, 2001).

Current Policies Affecting Engagement in Employment

Government policies affect older Americans' employment in both direct and indirect ways. Certain policies create explicit economic incentives or disincentives for employers to hire older workers and for older employees to seek and/or maintain employment. Other policies manipulate the job market, set the tone of work environments, and guide institutional rules for employers, which in turn influence work decisions of and opportunities for the older worker. Government intervention in elderly employment can be summarized into the following four categories: (1) providing or changing availability and sufficiency of retirement income, (2) providing financial (dis-) incentives to work, (3) offering direct employment services, and, (4) guiding workplace policies (Kim, 2003).

Retirement Income. Social Security and pension benefits are the key sources of retirement income for many workers; and these benefits influence the work decision of older people. Indeed, the availability of this income has made it possible for workers to terminate employment. Until recently, there existed a strong work disincentive in the Social Security program because of two major provisions—"delayed retirement credit" and the "earnings test" (Shelton, 2000; Uccello, 1998). Under the law, individuals were eligible to receive full benefits at age 65, which is the "normal" retirement age. For those who chose to continue to work and delayed benefit receipt beyond age 65, there was a "delayed retirement credit" of 3% per year as of 1990. This award of 3% credit for delay of benefit receipt was less than actuarially fair and lowered expected lifetime benefits. Thus, it created a strong financial disincentive for delaying benefit receipt (in other words, a strong financial incentive to retire at the normal age) (Burkhauser & Quinn, 1997; Herz & Philip, 1989; Kollmann, 2000). Under the provision of the earnings test, when a Social Security beneficiary continued to work and earned income exceeded a certain threshold, called the "exempt amount," a reduced benefit was paid to the beneficiary. In this way, the law maintained a further incentive to retire or withdraw from paid employment (Burkhauser & Quinn, 1997; Herz & Philip, 1989; Kollmann, 2000)

Recently, as the two provisions had been under attack, several amendments have removed some of the disincentive. Recent legislation in the year 2000 abolished the earnings limits for some older workers. For workers who reach normal retirement age, benefits are not reduced regardless of the amount of earnings. Moreover, the delayed retirement credit will increase from 3% until it reaches 8% per year in 2008 (Senior Citizen's Freedom to Work Act of 2000).

The private pension system is the other major retirement income source, and it greatly affects work decisions for those who have pension benefits. Private pension plans are regulated under the federal law, the Employee Retirement Income Security Act (ERISA) of 1974, which sets minimum standards to protect workers. Currently, there are two types of private pension plans: defined benefit plans and defined contribution plans. Defined benefit plans allow benefits earned after the normal retirement age to accrue at a slower rate; thus, benefits are age related, and the system discourages working into older ages. In addition, as defined benefit plans commonly contain early retirement benefits, they tend to provide strong financial disincentive to work beyond certain ages. On the other hand, under defined contribution plans, benefit accumulation is more age neutral, and voluntary contributions are allowed in most cases. Thus, defined contribution plans do not discourage work as strongly as defined benefit plans do. Historically, defined benefit plans were the predominant form of employer-provided pension systems, but there is a recent trend toward defined contribution plans. Thus, work disincentives are being further reduced (American Association of Retired Persons, 2001; Burkhauser & Quinn, 1997; Herz & Philip, 1989).

Tax Incentives and Disincentives. The Earned Income Tax Credit (EITC) was created in 1975 to help offset the burden of increasing Social Security payroll taxes for low-wage workers. The credits are available to lower-income taxpayers who have at least some earnings from employment during the year. The amount of credit is computed based on number of children in the family and level of earning. Despite the success of the EITC program in both reducing poverty and promoting work, it only covers workers who are under the age 65. As the program was originally designed for families with children, it excludes older workers from its benefits. This means that, while government provides a financial incentive to work for most Americans as a way of wage subsidy, it does not provide any incentives for older Americans (Earned Income Credit, 2003; Gary & Quinn, 2000).

Taxation of Social Security benefits also can be a work disincentive to older workers. Social Security benefits are taxable, and taxation occurs when beneficiaries' incomes exceed certain levels. For example, a married couple with an income of more than $32,000 is subject to taxes on up to 85% of their Social Security benefits. This means that an older person receives less after-tax Social Security income as their total incomes increase. Thus, the taxation of Social Security benefits discourages work effort after age 65 years of age (Gary & Quinn, 2000; U.S. House and Representatives, 2000).

Employment Services. The Senior Community Service Employment Program (SCSEP) was established under Title V of the Old Americans Act of 1965. It provides employment services for part-time jobs, specifically targeting low-income individuals who are aged 55 and older and unemployed. Individuals who are 60 years old or older have priority for the work opportunities provided under the act. By fostering part-time job opportunities in community service activities, the program intends to promote individual economic self-sufficiency and, ultimately, increases the number of participants placed in unsubsidized employment in the public and private sectors. The program, thus, assists older workers in obtaining regular unsubsidized jobs through counseling, job search assistance, support services, and a limited amount of job training (Chao & Fiala, 2001; Samorodov, 1999).

When the Older American Act was amended in 2000, it strengthened the connection between SCSEP and the Workforce Investment Act (WIA) of 1998 to provide older individuals with easier access to appropriate services while minimizing duplication of services. One of the objectives of the WIA is to increase the employment, retention, and occupational skill of the program participants. As WIA includes SCSEP as a required partner in the delivery system, it ensures employment-related services to older workers (Nightingale, 1998). Throughout its history, SCSEP has served some of the most disadvantaged older adults, particularly those with poverty incomes, limited educational attainment, and minorities (Chao & Fiala, 2001; Nightingale, 1998).

Guidelines Against Discrimination. Discriminatory practices can play a role in forcing older workers from the workforce. The Age Discrimination in Employment Act (ADEA) was enacted in 1967 to (1) prohibit arbitrary age discrimination in hiring and other employment practices, (2) promote the employment of older workers based on ability rather than age, and (3) help employers and employees find ways to meet problems arising from the impact of age on employment (American Association of Retired Persons, 2001). Under the law, individuals 40 years old and older are protected from age discrimination. The law generally prohibits employers from establishing maximum hiring or mandatory retirement ages for their workers. According to the law, any individuals aggrieved by illegal discriminatory practices at workplaces are entitled to bring a civil action. The Equal Employment Opportunity Commission (EEOC) has the power to make investigations.

Deteriorating health conditions and physical impairments present challenges for some older adults to stay employed or return to work. Older persons constitute more than 60% of population with disabilities, and the aging of the American workforce is likely to increase the number of employees with disabilities (American Association of Retired Persons, 2001). Thus, disability policies can affect employment of the elderly. The Americans with Disabilities Act (ADA) of 1990 was created primarily to protect disabled people from employment discrimination. The act requires employers to make reasonable accommodations to allow disabled employees to perform the essential functions of the job or to assist the employees in the application process if necessary. It also contains requirements for elimination of physical barriers to access (EEOC, 1997). The impact of ADA on older adults' decision to work may not be substantial because it affects only those who have disabilities and manipulates work environments only indirectly (Burkhauser & Quinn, 1997).

Effects of Engagement

A substantial body of literature over the years documents a positive relationship between employment and well-being, even when health and financial status have been controlled (Conner, Dorfman, & Thompkins, 1985; Mathers & Schofield, 1998). Methodological limitations have weakened causal conclusions in most of this work because health and mental health factors are both causes and effects of employment status (Kasl & Jones, 2000).

A large longitudinal study confirms the positive relationship between employment and health. Gallo, Bradley, Siegal, and Kasl (2000) studied older adults working in plants over a 2-year period. Those who were involuntarily laid off during the observation period had poorer physical functioning and mental health outcomes, controlling for prejob-loss health status, labor income, and net worth. The strongest negative effects were on mental health outcomes. Furthermore, those older adults who regained employment had improved health and mental health outcomes at subsequent observations. These researchers conclude that late-stage job loss has important consequences for well-being, including mental health, physical health, and financial outcomes. Gallo and colleagues point out that older workers are displaced from jobs more than younger adults; thus, these negative effects need to be considered as part of any counseling or relocation services offered.

The mechanisms by which employment contributes to well-being are not thoroughly understood. Mor-Barak, Scharlach, Birba, and Sokolov (1992) posited that for older adults, employment is related to larger social networks and, through this relationship, to better perceived health. They tested three social networks factors (family, friends, and confidant relationships) and found that employment was related to the friendship component. Mor-Barak (1995) further explored the meaning of work for older individuals and found that the generativity factor—that is, viewing work as a way to teach, train, and share skills with the younger generation—is particularly important to older adults. Aquino, Russell, Cutrona, and Altmaier (1996) considered paid and unpaid (volunteer) work and tested the hypothesis that employment is associated with social support and companionship, controlling for age, income, and mental and physical health. They found that the number of paid hours is related directly to life satisfaction (not through social support). On the other hand, volunteer work is related to increased social support, and social support is related to life satisfaction. In sum, paid work has a direct relationship to life satisfaction, whereas unpaid work (volunteering) has an indirect relationship to life satisfaction.

The positive effects of employment seem to be conditioned by various factors. Herzog, House, & Morgan (1991) found that older people whose work patterns reflect their personal preferences report higher levels of physical and psychological well-being than do people whose involvement in work is not under their control due to involuntary retirement or other factors. Rushing, Ritter, and Burton (1992) reported that being employed is a protective factor for mortality for Whites; whereas Blacks, whether employed or unemployed, are at greater risk for poorer health. Gallo and colleagues (2000) documented that older workers and unmarried workers have worse mental health outcomes in face of involuntary job loss.

In a review of the literature on job loss, retirement, and health, Kasl and Jones (2000) concluded that unemployment is associated with 20%–30% excess in mortality in most studies, that the impact of unemployment on morbidity is evident, and that unemployment clearly increases psychological distress. They separated their discussion of unemployment from that of retirement because these are two different phenomena. Retirement involves being unemployed but, in most cases, one enters retirement in a voluntary and planned on-time way. Of course, retirement can be entered involuntarily or off-time, and it is suggested that this trajectory may be associated with negative outcomes, yet there is only minimal evidence to support this (Ekerdt, 1995). They (Kasl & Jones, 2000) concluded that the research supports no adverse outcome of retirement per se and that variations in postretirement outcomes most likely reflect preretirement status in physical health, social and leisure activities, well-being, and life satisfaction.

In sum, the trend toward early retirement has leveled off and there are signs that older adults are working longer. The productive activity of paid employment is, in general, associated with increased health and mental health of older workers. However, there are certain subgroups of older adults who do not benefit from such positive outcomes, including workers who are not in positions that reflect their preference. In addition, some subpopulations do not benefit as much from employment, such as Black older adults. Changing employment policies are reducing disincentives to retire early, but despite legal protection, older adults experience discrimination in the workforce. It has been suggested that older adults are the "shock absorbers" for the changing American economy, and they are vulnerable to layoffs, inadequate salaries, and discrimination (Kaye & Alexander, 1995). Despite solid evidence that older adults are valuable employees, Mor-Barak & Wilson (in press) conclude that the workplace remains by and large a hostile environment for older adults as a result of overt and covert age discrimination.

VOLUNTEERING

Current Levels of Engagement

Elders are actively engaged in their communities and volunteer work (Fisher, Day, & Collier, 1998), and it appears that volunteering in later life is on the rise. A variety of surveys have shown that there was a substantial increase in volunteering by older adults in the last quarter of the 20th century (Chamber, 1993). The proportion of older persons volunteering varies greatly from survey to survey.[2] Currently, about 44% of people aged 55 and over volunteered 4.4 hours per week on average in the past year (Independent Sector, 2002). Totally, 26.4 million older volunteers contributed approximately 5.6 billion hours, at the value of 77.2 billion dollars (Independent Sector, 2002).

There are variations among different age brackets in volunteering status. It is estimated that 50.3% of people aged 55 to 64, 46.6% of aged 65 to 74, and 43.0% aged 75 years and over participated in volunteer work in 1998 (U.S. Bureau of the Census, 2001). The volunteer rates for these three age groups have increased by 3.3, 3.6, and 6.6%, respectively, since 1994 (U.S. Bureau of the Census, 1996). The figures are consistent with the findings in current studies, which document relatively high rates of volunteering among the younger olds, while finding reduced rates among those over 75 years of age (Caro & Bass, 1995). However, volunteering by elders ages 75 and over has increased at the highest rate among the three groups. Although the volunteer rate is lower among older generations than the younger, older volunteers devote more hours once they are involved. According to the most recent Current Population Survey, volunteers age 65 and over contributed most to volunteer activities with a median of 96 hours during the year of 2001, whereas volunteers age 25 to 34 spent a median of 34 hours (Bureau of Labor Statistics, 2002).

Most evidence indicates that age is not significantly related to volunteer hours across the adult life span until very late in life (Herzog, Kahn, Morgan, Jackson, & Antonucci, 1989). Other demographic characteristics such as gender, race, and marital status are not strongly associated with volunteering in later life; but these findings are inconsistent (Fisher & Schaffer, 1993). For example, Caro and Bass (1995) found that female seniors were more likely to volunteer, while other studies do not reveal that gender makes a significant difference in volunteer status and amount (Chambre, 1984; Cnaan & Cascio, 1999; Herzog & Morgan, 1993; Musick, Herzog, & House; 1999; Warburton, Brocque, & Rosenman, 1998). In comparison, socioeconomic status, represented by education, occupation, and income, is related to volunteering (Sundeen, 1992). Education is the most significant factor (Caro & Bass, 1995; Fisher & Schaffer, 1993). Generally, higher socioeconomic status predicts more volunteer participation (Smith, 1994). It is found that white-collar workers are one-and-a-half times more likely to volunteer than are blue-collar workers (Warburton et al., 1998). According to a rational choice perspective, level of volunteering is inversely related to income because opportunity costs increase as wages rise (Wilson, 2000); yet, this perspective may not be applicable to older volunteers, whose income has no effect on the overall hours of volunteering (Gallagher, 1994). Volunteering also is found to be associated with employment status, health, and social integration. Among older adults, part-time workers are more likely to volunteer than are full-time workers and retirees (Fisher & Schaffer, 1993; Herzog & Morgan, 1993). In addition, older people in good health and with more social integration are more likely to engage in volunteer work (Herzog & Morgan, 1993; Okun, 1993; Thoits & Hewitt, 2001).

Current Policies Affecting Engagement

The tax code of the United States calls for deductions of expenses related to volunteering. The Internal Revenue Service's *Charitable Contributions Publication 526* declares that volunteers can claim a deduction for mileage, parking, paper, uniforms, and so on if the organizations do not compensate them for the expenses incurred in volunteering (Service Leader, 1999). Beyond this taxation policy, other federal initiatives to support volunteering involve the creation of programs. Most public policy that affects older volunteers stems from two statutes: the Domestic Volunteer Service Act of 1973 and the National and Community Service Act of 1990, as well as their amendments (USA Freedom Corps, 2002). The National and Community Service Act authorizes several programs; for example, AmeriCorp, Learn and Serve America, the National Civilian Community Corps, and the Point of Light Foundation. The Domestic Volunteer Service Act authorizes the Volunteer in Service to America (VISTA) and National Senior Volunteer Corps. In addition, the USA Freedom Corps has recently been established to expand public volunteering and service opportunities for all American citizens (USA Freedom Corps, 2002).

AmeriCorps is the largest program to promote national and community service. AmeriCorps is geared toward youth, and fewer than 3% of AmeriCorps volunteers are over the age of 60 (Freedman, 2002). One of its components, the National Civilian Community Corps, exclusively recruits youth between the ages of 18 to 24 (Abt Associates Inc., 2001). It has been pointed out that incentive structures favor youth, and there are calls to modify program structure to increase multigenerational participation (Freedman, 2002). Learn and Serve America is strongly biased toward youth in its organization through schools, colleges, and universities (Center for Human Resources, 1999). Elderhostel has developed a form of learn and serve for seniors that can empower older volunteers and increase their connections with both the consumers of the service provided and the volunteer projects (Carden, 2001).

Specifically related to volunteering by older adults, the National Senior Service Corps, under the administration of the Corporation for National Service, consists of the Foster Grandparent Program, the Senior Companion Program, and the Retired and Senior Volunteer Program (RSVP) (Westat, 1998). The Foster Grandparent Program and the Senior Companion Program have the same eligibility requirements; namely, Foster Grandparents and Senior Companions must be 60 years or above, with an income of 125% or135% of the Department of Health and Human Services Poverty Guidelines (Senior Corps, 2002a). According to the current requirements, participants in both programs must serve on average 20 hours per week and must receive small stipends of $2.65 per hour (USA Freedom Corps, 2002). Revisions are currently being discussed, with proposals to enhance Senior Corps through lowering the age eligibility from 60 to 55 for all programs, removing the income eligibility limitations, adding new flexibility in service scope and time commitment, creating a senior scholarship program, requiring accountability, and increasing budget (USA Freedom Corps, 2002). It is hoped that older Americans will be provided with expanded opportunities to participate in community and volunteering services under the Citizen Service Act of 2002, which reforms the Corporation for National and Community Service (USA Freedom Corps, 2002).

Senior Companions matches volunteers to frail adults who need assistance and friendship (Aguirre International, 2001a). In the year of 2001, approximately 15,500 Senior Companions provided services to 61, 300 clients with a total of over 13.6 million hours (Senior Corps, 2002b). About half (49%) of the participants were 65 to 74 years old; 31% fell into the age bracket of 75 to 84; 15% range from 60 to 64 years; and 5% of Senior Companions were 85 years and over (Senior Corps, 2002b).

Foster Grandparents serve as mentors, tutors, and caregivers for children and youth with special needs in such community organizations as schools, hospitals, Head Start, and youth centers (Senior Corps, 2002c). During the year of 2001, about 30,200 Foster Grandparents served over 275,000 children and youth with a total of more than 27.3 million hours (Senior Corps, 2002c). The percentages of age groups involved in the service are quite similar to those in Senior Companion: 14% aged 60 to 64 years; 49% aged 65 to 74; 32% aged 75 to 84; and 5% aged 85 years and above (Senior Corps, 2002c).

Unlike the Senior Companion and the Foster Grandparent policies that provide in-cash incentives, the RSVP matches adults aged 55 and over to volunteer positions aimed at their communities' needs (Senior Corps, 2002d). RSVP volunteers serve 4 hours per week on average, without stipend under the current requirement, while it is proposed that they be provided with an allowance for a longer period of time in service (USA Freedom Corps, 2002). In the year of 2001, about 480,000 volunteers devoted approximately 77 million hours in 766 projects within 7 emphasis areas: health and nutrition, human needs services, education, environment, public safety, community and economic development, and leadership (Aguirre International, 2001b; Senior Corps 2002d). Among the volunteers, 4% were aged 55 to 59 years, 11% aged 60 to 64, 38% aged 65 to 74, 37% aged 75 to 84, and 10% aged 85 and older (Senior Corps, 2002d).

As part of Foreign Relations and Intercourse Act, the Peace Corps was initiated in 1961 with aims to help the people in interested countries and help promote mutual understanding between Americans and other people (Peace Corps, n.d.). Currently, about

7,000 Peace Corps volunteers are serving in 70 countries, working in sectors of education, health, environment, business, agriculture, and others (Peace Corps, 2002a). Volunteers aged 50 and over account for 7% of the total members, and the oldest volunteer is 82 years old (Peace Corps, 2002a). Financial benefits received by volunteers include a monthly living allowance, transportation, medical health coverage and insurance plan, loan deferment or partial cancellation, reimbursement of $6,075, and vacation (Peace Corps, 2002b).

Started in 1964 by the Small Business Administration, the Service Corps of Retired Executives (SCORE) aims to engage retired business executives in counseling and mentoring services to the public without charge (Chambre, 1993; The Catalog of Federal Domestic Assistance, n.d.). Since its inception, approximately 11,500 SCORE volunteers have helped 4.2 million people start or develop their own business (The Catalog of Federal Domestic Assistance, n.d.).

Caro and Morris (2003) point out that the discussion of senior volunteer programs often begins and ends with federal initiatives. Indeed, the programs reviewed have been very successful in engaging citizens in service activities; but they have been criticized for limiting participation of older adults. Further, senior volunteer initiatives have been criticized for failing to encourage innovation in the development of service programs soliciting older adult volunteers (Freedman, 2002). Freedman (1999) described how older adults have taken the development of meaningful opportunities into their own hands through the creation of programs providing vital health and educational services to communities across the country. These programs solicit older adults for their time and talent and target some of our society's most pressing issues: failing schools, environmental degradation, youth drug abuse, and child maltreatment. Most financial support comes from foundations and private/corporate contributions, with some partnerships with state or local governments. Also, some receive demonstration money from federal sources (Morrow-Howell, Carden, & Sherraden, in press).

Effects of Engagement

There is extensive literature that associates volunteering with improved well-being outcomes for the older adult. Yet, most of the research is cross-sectional in design and does not allow us to conclude that volunteering causes positive outcomes. Indeed, it is documented that healthier, more educated, higher income people

volunteer (Fisher & Schaffer, 1993), and these variables are con-
founded with volunteering in these associative analyses. There are
only a few older studies that achieved quasiexperimental designs
and demonstrated that older adults experienced positive gains from
volunteering (SRA Technologies, 1985; Litigation Support Services,
1984). For example, over a 3-year period, Foster Grandparents were
compared to those older adults who wanted to volunteer but
remained on a waitlist. For the volunteers, there were gains in mental health and social resources; while for nonvolunteers, there were
declines on these measures.

There are a several newer longitudinal analyses that support the
positive impact of volunteering on older adults' health and mental
health. For example, over a 30-year period, women involved in volunteer activities retained higher levels of functional ability (Moen,
Dempster-McClain, & Williams, 1992). Analyses showed that women,
who occupied multiple roles, including volunteer roles, had higher
levels of social integration and better health. Also, over an 8-year
period, older adults who volunteered had lower mortality rates than
did nonvolunteers (Musick, Herzog, & House, 1999), even after
controlling for health, socioeconomic status, and social integration.
Further analyses on the same longitudinal data set show that older
adults who volunteered report higher levels of self-rated health,
higher life satisfaction, increased function, and lower levels of depression; and that some of these effects are greater than those attained by
younger volunteers (Morrow-Howell, Hinterlong, Rozario, & Tang,
2003; Van Willigen, 2000). Some studies suggest that more disadvantaged elders, for example, elders who are socially isolated or physically impaired, benefit more from undertaking volunteer activities;
but the evidence is mixed (Fengler, 1984; Musick et al., 1999; Van
Willigen, 2000; Morrow-Howell et al., 2003).

Scholars have speculated on the reasons that volunteering seems
to improve health outcomes; but there is now solid evidence that
tells us why volunteering is good for older adults. Ideas include
increased feelings of usefulness and self-esteem (Hunter & Linn,
1980-1981); role replacement (Chambre, 1987); reduction in social
isolation (Moen et al., 1992); provision of structure and opportunity for meaningful involvement (Freedman, 1994); increases in
resources, power, and prestige associated with role enhancement
(Musick et al., 1999). Of course, the reciprocal relationships of volunteering and health make the development of causal knowledge
very challenging. In a recent analysis, Thoits and Hewitt (2001)

document the reciprocal relationship between volunteer hours and well-being. They show that well-being facilitates volunteer involvement and that volunteer involvement subsequently augments well-being. Morrow-Howell and colleagues (2003) suggest that we have accumulated enough evidence that volunteering is good for older adults and that from a public health perspective it makes sense to maximize involvement.

In sum, volunteering among older adults is not only alive and well, it is growing. Future generations are more likely to come forward to serve in even larger numbers (Peter D. Hart Research Associates, 1999). Engagement in volunteering appears to have positive effects on health, mental health, and life satisfaction. Further, the benefits most likely accrue to both the volunteer and the community being served. Public policy has contributed to the engagement of older adults in volunteer roles through the creation of service programs; but these programs are biased toward youth. Some programs geared specifically to older Americans restrict access to low-income older adults. Innovative and inclusive policy initiatives are needed to maximize the engagement of older adults in volunteer roles.

CAREGIVING

Current Levels of Engagement

Contrary to the popular belief that older adults are care recipients, numerous older adults are care providers for dependent relatives (Doty, 1995; Tennstedt, 1999; Wagner, 1997). Older adults provide care to their very old parents, dependent adult children, grandchildren, siblings, relatives, friends and neighbors; but spousal caregiving is the most prevalent (Bass & Caro, 2001). Using a sample of persons aged 65 and over in the 1991 Commonwealth Fund Survey, Doty (1995) reports that 26% of those aged 65 and over and 22% of those aged 75 and over are involved in providing assistance to sick and disabled people. She emphasizes that this proportion is twice the proportion of aged 65 and over needing care. In addition, about 15% of participants in the survey indicated that they provided assistance to disabled people more than 20 hours a week, and this proportion was 7% of those aged 65 and over. Based on a sample of the 1989 National Long-term Care Survey, it is found that 53% of primary caregivers for dependent elderly were aged 65 and over (Doty, 1995).

While younger caregivers are dominantly female, gender differences are not noticeable among older caregivers (Doty, 1995; Tennstedt, 1999). Among older caregivers, there are as many male spousal caregivers as female spousal caregivers, and male spousal caregivers are reported to help their care recipients with the activities of daily living (ADL) tasks similarly to female spousal caregivers.

Current Policies Affecting Engagement

Caregiving policies are categorized into direct in-cash assistance, indirect in-cash assistance, in-kind assistance programs, and regulation (Rozario, 2000). Direct in-cash assistance policies and programs that pay informal caregivers include Medicaid personal care waivers, cash and counseling demonstration projects, and Veterans Administration (VA) housebound aid and attendance allowance (Rozario, 2000). Medicaid personal care waiver programs enable states to establish programs that pay informal caregivers. Michigan, Texas, and California have such programs, wherein informal caregivers (of care recipients who are eligible for Medicaid and meet disability criteria) can be paid for their services (Stone & Keigher, 1994). The informal caregivers of this program include children, siblings, or other family members, whereas spousal caregivers are excluded. Given that state funding is involved in these Medicaid programs, benefit levels and funding source differ from state to state (Linsk, Keigher, Simon-Rusinowitz, & England, 1992).

Cash and counseling demonstration programs provide functionally impaired older adults with cash allowances and counseling (in the form of education, support, etc.) to arrange and pay for the services they need (Rozario, 2000). This Medicaid-related program is operating on a demonstration basis in Arkansas, Florida, New Jersey, Oregon, and Colorado (U.S. Department of Health and Human Services, 2002). In these programs, cash allowance can be used to hire caregivers, including family members. Older adults with disabilities are more likely to utilize this program, compared to younger adults with disabilities (Foster, Brown, Carlson, Philips, & Schore, 2000). As this program mainly focuses on care recipients' control over care arrangements, the impact of older caregivers is not yet known. The VA housebound aid and attendance allowance program offers cash allowance to low-income disabled veterans (including surviving spouses) who need personal care. This allowance can be used to pay for the services of their informal caregivers (Grana & Yamashiro, 1987; Rozario, 2000).

Indirect in-cash assistance programs offer tax credits that informal caregivers can claim for formal caregiving expenses. Indirect in-cash assistance programs include federal child and dependent care tax credit and dependent care assistance plans. The federal child and dependent care tax credit program allows an employed individual to claim credit for coresiding dependents, including mentally or physically dependent persons (spouses are not excluded). The amount of credit given is based on the amount of work-related dependent care expenses the person paid to a formal care provider. The dependent care assistance program provides tax deductions for formal caregiving expenses, and it can be claimed by employers or employed caregivers (Internal Revenue Service, 2001). Both programs are for employed caregivers, and, hence, caregivers who are not employed (most older caregivers) do not benefit.

In-kind assistance programs include the National Family Caregiver Support program and respite and support programs provided by the Veterans Health Administration (VHA). The National Family Caregiver Support program was established by the enactment of the Older Americans Act Amendments of 2000 (Public Law 106-501). It was modeled after successful state long term care programs in California, New Jersey, Wisconsin, Pennsylvania, and other states (Administration on Aging, n.d.). The program provides the following five basic services for family caregivers: (1) information to caregivers about available services, (2) assistance to caregivers in gaining access to services, (3) individual counseling, organization of support groups, and caregiver training, (4) respite care, and (5) supplemental services. Eligible persons for this program include (1) family caregivers of older adults and (2) grandparents and relative caregivers of children not older than age 18 (including grandparents who are sole caregivers of grandchildren and those individuals who are affected by mental retardation or who have developmental disabilities). The Administration on Aging (n.d.) reports that this program was funded at $125 million in fiscal year 2001 and approximately $113 million has been allocated to states through a congressionally-mandated formula that is based on a proportionate share of the population age 70 and older. This program requires all states, working in partnership with area agencies on aging and local community-service providers, to have the five basic services for family caregivers.

U.S. Department of Veterans Affairs (n.d.) indicates that VHA offers up to 30 days per year of respite care services to veterans. VA nursing homes and intermediate care units have designated respite beds, and many VHA facilities offer contract respite services in community nursing homes for veterans with special needs. The respite care services allow caregivers to take a break from caregiving responsibilities. VHA also offers caregiver support programs, including facilitated support groups, information and education, and counseling services.

The Family and Medical Leave Act (FMLA), administered by the U.S. Department of Labor, entitles eligible employees[3] to take up to 12 weeks of unpaid, job-protected leave in a 12-month period for, among other things, providing care to an immediate family member (spouse, child, or parent) with a serious health condition. A covered employer is required to maintain group health insurance coverage for an employee on FMLA leave whenever such insurance was provided before the leave was taken and on the same terms as if the employee had continued to work. Upon return from FMLA leave, an employee must be restored to the employee's original job or to an equivalent job with equivalent pay, benefits, and other terms and conditions of employment. The Commission on Family and Medical Leave (1996) shows that about 55% of U.S. workers are eligible for the FMLA leave, and the FMLA utilization rate among eligible workers is estimated to be at least 2%. About 10% of the leaves are taken by older employees to provide care to an ill parent or spouse. Although 47% of leave takers have full wage replacement, the oldest and youngest employees, nonsalaried workers, and nonunion workers are less likely to receive wage replacement (Commission on Family and Medical Leave, 1996).

Effects of Engagement in Caregiving

There is abundant evidence, from almost 20 years of research, that caregiving for a dependent relative can negatively impact a person's physical health, mental health, and financial status (Cantor, 1983; George & Gwyther, 1986; Wilcox & King, 1999). Of course, a great deal of the research involves nonrepresentative samples and does not involve comparison groups (Marks, 1998); but the association of caregiving for dependent elders with negative outcomes seems undeniable. Caregivers report higher levels of depression (Strawbridge, Wallhagen et al., 1997); worse self-perceived health (Schulz, Visintainer, & Williamson, 1990); more physical health symptoms (Wallsten, 2000); increased physical decline (White-Means & Thorton, 1996) and worse mental health (Tennestedt, Cafferata, & Sullivan, 1992).

Biological studies have documented that caregivers have altered immune function (Esterling et al., 1994). Cardiovascular reactivity and blood pressure elevations are increased under stress in caregivers as compared to controls; also it is documented that caregivers have metabolic changes compared to non-caregivers, including insulin levels, glucose levels, and weight gain (Vitaliano et al., 1996a/b). The impact of the physical and psychological stress of caregiving leads to higher levels of medical help-seeking and medication use than noncaregiving control groups as well as higher incidence of physical illness (Schulz et al., 1995). Indeed, Schulz and Beach (1999) document that among coresidential spousal caregivers, caregivers reporting caregiving strain had mortality risks 63% higher than did noncaregivers, after controlling for health status and other sociodemographic factors.

Zarit, Gaugler, and Jarrott (1999) remind us that caregiver burden results from care-related stressors, mediated by contextual variables and available resources, and that individuals vary greatly in their response to caregiving. Townsend and his colleagues (1989) used longitudinal data to document the great variability in adaptation to caregiving. Sources of variability have been studied quite a great deal. Most studies report that women experienced more negative outcomes than did men (Yee & Schulz, 2000), and that spousal caregivers were more strongly impacted than were caregivers with other relationships (Neal, Ingersoll-Dayton, & Starrels, 1997). Caregivers experiencing health problems reported more negative outcomes than did nonill caregivers (Bull, 1990). Coping style and social support have been widely tested as moderators (Intrieri & Rapp, 1994). Age and prior resources moderated the effect of caregiving on well-being (Moen, Robison, & Dempster-McClain, 1995). Caregivers who found meaning in the role were less depressed; finding meaning meant that they held positive beliefs about the caregiving situation and the self as caregiver (Noonan & Tennstedt (1997). When caregivers perceived a more positive relationship with the care recipient (described as "mutuality" by the researchers), caregivers reported less burden (Robinson, 1990).

There are examples of null findings in the literature, as well as work that highlights some positive aspects of caregiving. For example, Seltzer and Li (2000) found no difference between caregivers and noncaregivers in personal growth and depression. Strawbridge and his colleagues (1997) found no difference in physical health outcomes between caregivers and noncaregivers over a 20-year period.

Moen, Robison, and Dempster-McClain (1995) found no direct effects of caregiving or duration of caregiving on well-being measures. Marks (1998) studied midlife caregivers and noncaregivers and found few negative effects of caregiving on positive dimensions of psychological wellness (purpose in life, self-acceptance, environmental mastery). He assessed work-family conflict differences between caregivers and noncaregivers. After controlling for conflicts experienced in the workplace due to caregiving, the negative effects of caregiving were attenuated. Further, when work-family conflicts were controlled, some positive effects of caregiving were revealed, for example, more positive relations, more purpose in life, more personal growth. These researchers conclude that workplace policies and environments can reduce work-family conflict for caregivers and thereby reduce the negative effects of caregiving and allow the psychological benefits of caregiving to emerge.

Satisfaction is the most common positive outcome associated with caregiving, and caregivers generally articulate more rewards associated with the role than problems (Walker, Shin, & Bird, 1990). Potential benefits reported in the literature include enhanced sense of self-efficacy, improved relationship with care recipient, congruence with one's religious or ethical principles, sense of purpose and meaning, and reassurance that care recipient is getting optimal care (Kramer, 1997; Scharlach, 1994).

It has been suggested that additional productive roles in addition to caregiver may lead to beneficial effects on well-being outcomes (Moen et al., 1989, 1992). The positive aspects of combining caregiving and work have been documented (Scharlach, 1994). Tennstedt and colleagues (1992) found that nonemployed caregivers were more depressed than were employed caregivers. Spitze, Logan, Joseph, and Lee (1994), studying a large sample of midlife men and women, found that combining employment with caregiving related to less distress for men. However, for women, there was no effect of combining employment and caregiving. A majority of employed caregivers view their work as a break from caregiving (Lechner & Gupta, 1996). Further, it is proposed that employment provides resources that maintain the mental health of caregivers (Faison, Faria, & Frank, 1999).

In sum, more older adults are caregivers than care recipients. Spousal caregivers provide care in compromised health conditions and on fixed incomes. The current policies supporting older caregivers are limited, as most policies and programs are directed toward the care recipient. Although they may indirectly benefit the caregiver, policies fail to directly recognize and reward caregivers for their services. For example, spousal caregivers are not eligible for direct in-cash assistance under Medicaid waiver programs, tax credits are limited to coresiding dependents, and respite programs do not go far enough in providing needed support. The National Family Caregiver Support is new, and outcomes are yet unknown; but the amount of money that eventually reaches the local level is quite small (Administration on Aging, n.d.). The vast majority of research regarding outcomes on caregiving uses a stress and coping framework to document the negative outcomes associated with this extremely important role in later life. However, Kramer (1997) argues that research has not focused on understanding the positive impacts of caregiving and that this lack of attention has skewed perceptions of the caregiving experience. She points out that caregivers experience both positive and negative emotions, and we need to understand the gains of caregiving if we are truly to support and develop program for caregivers. Clearly, public policy initiatives need to find better ways to develop programs that create conditions of engagement that maximize positive outcomes or at least reduce negative outcomes for the caregiver.

MAXIMIZING POTENTIAL THROUGH INSTITUTIONAL CAPACITY

In this chapter, we demonstrate that older adults have high levels of engagement in the productive activities of working, volunteering, and caregiving. In a secondary analysis of a large longitudinal data set following people over the age of 60 for 8 years, Hinterlong (2002) demonstrates that older adults averaged 563 hours (SD = 854.8) of productive activity in an average of 2.04 roles at the first observation. At the last observation, these older adults, now 8 years older, contributed 269.7 hrs. (SD = 681.6) in 1.83 roles. This analysis demonstrates that older adults continue in productive activities, maintaining involvement in productive roles while reducing time in these roles. Caro and Bass (1992) conclude that more than a quarter of the elderly population work, more than a quarter volunteer, more than a quarter provide assistance to a disabled person, and 40% help children and grandchildren.

We also demonstrate that social policies exist that affect older adults' experiences in these productive roles. Employment policies are changing in favor of extending longer working lives for the American work force, but age discrimination still limits the effectiveness of new laws. Few policies affect volunteering beyond federally-funded service programs, and there is a bias toward youth service in these initiatives. Despite the huge cost savings to society and the heavy price paid by older caregivers, policies that directly support older caregivers are limited.

We suggest that social policies and programs need to be examined and changed to increase opportunities for work and volunteering among older adults and to further encourage and reward older adults in their difficult jobs as caregivers. The longevity revolution has created a reservoir of individual capacity. Older adults in this society are healthier, more financially secure, and not only are they able, but they desire, to continue to make contributions to their families and communities. We proposed that we need to increase the institutional capacity of our society to engage the potential of these older adults. Our society has experienced the power of public policy to affect decisions made about later life (e.g., Social Security and retirement). Sherraden, Morrow-Howell, Hinterlong, and Rozario (2001, p. 278) ask, "What would be the public policy for productivity through the life course? What would be the programs, regulations, and tax laws that defined this policy? And what institutional structures would these policies create?" Institutional capacity refers to the ability of social institutions, like businesses, public and private agencies, churches, legal institutions, and social or civic clubs to create and promote productive roles for older adults. Institutions can offer information, incentives, and on-going support for older adults in these roles, and these structural variables are likely to affect the amount of engagement and the outcomes of engagement for the older adults as well as for society (Morrow-Howell, Hinterlong, Rozario, & Tang, 2003). That is, social structures may explain a large part of the variance in productive behaviors, as suggested in the works of Bass and Caro (2001), and as reflected in the "structural lag" theory of Matilda White Riley (Riley, Kahn, & Foner, 1994). Riley and her colleagues also point out that institutions are to some extent created and changed by people, which means that policy and program innovations are possible.

Policy innovations that maximize the involvement of older adults in productive roles may contribute to public health; as there is enough evidence from related studies of health, mental health, and life satisfaction to conclude that, in general, engagement in productive roles of work and volunteering is beneficial to older adults. Although some beneficial psychological aspects of caregiving are documented, the very important role of caregiving to dependent elders is often related to negative health and mental health outcomes for the older caregiver. There is some support for the idea that multiple role involvement (or role enhancement) improves the well-being outcomes for caregivers, suggesting that combining work or volunteer roles with caregiving roles may enhance outcomes.

Some older persons may benefit from one type of productive engagement more than another. The type of productive involvement leading toward the most positive outcomes for the older adult depends on individual preferences, cultural preferences, and family circumstances. An older person may benefit from respite caregiving to engage in full- or part-time work; or the older employee may benefit from exchanging work involvement for caregiving activities. These exchanges between types of productive engagement highlight questions about transitions between types of productive engagement and about policies and organizational structures that provide choice to individuals for productive involvement (Morrow-Howell, Hinterlong, Sherraden, & Rozario, 2001). To improve the outcomes of caregiving, it will be important to test institutional structures that give caregivers a choice to move between work and caregiving or to do both simultaneously with less negative consequences.

Perhaps some individuals may benefit most from being involved in multiple productive activities. Involvement in multiple roles has been linked to better health and longevity outcomes. It has been suggested that, in later life, multiple role occupancy may protect people from role reduction (Berkman & Breslow, 1983; House, Landis, & Umberson, 1988; Moen, Dempster-McClain, & Williams, 1989). However, studies that consider the impact of multiple roles on well-being outcomes have, by in large, focused on middle-aged people (Dautzenberg, Diederiks, Philipson, & Tan, 1999). What are the effects of multiple roles for different age groups in later life? Do caregivers in their 60s or in their 70s fare better if they also have volunteer involvement or part-time work?

Related to type of productive involvement are the various socio-environmental conditions in which the activity takes place. These conditions very likely influence the outcomes experienced by the older individual engaged in work, volunteer, and caregiving roles. In regard to work, there are many new employment structures, like job sharing and bridge employment, that may affect the experience of working in later life. Rowe and Kahn (1998) suggest the introduction of the 4-hour work module to increase flexibility in work arrangements is a potential benefit to younger and older workers alike. Bass, Quinn, and Burkhauser (1995) suggest that new policies provide part-time employees with prorated benefits and reduce private health care costs for employers employing older workers. What impact will these organizational arrangements have on the older worker's well-being?

In regard to volunteering, well-being outcomes may be related to the organizational environment that the older adult experiences—the amount of socialization involved, the characteristics of the volunteer assignments, the extent to which constructive working relationships between workers and volunteers exists, and the various types of compensation or reimbursement or recognition given (Morris & Caro, 1996). In the area of caregiving, we need to understand the impact that public policies, like tax credits or "cash and counseling" programs,[4] have on caregiving outcomes. Other institutional structures that effect caregivers' physical health and mental health include the availability and affordability of formal services to assist with the caregiving tasks, laws affecting job security, and company policies that effect eldercare (Gonyea, 1997; Hooyman & Gonyea, 1995).

Policy and program development will be challenged by the probability that *individual choice* is an important mediator in the relationship between productive involvement and well-being outcomes (Sherraden, Morrow-Howell, Hinterlong, & Rozario, 2001). Individual preference and choice are likely important ingredients in maximizing positive outcomes. These constructs are likely shaped by culture, gender, social class, and life experience. Further, given that there is a fixed quantity of time, energy, and commitment available (Goode, 1960), we need to further understand the optimal balance of time in productive roles. What about leisure time? Survey research indicates that older adults want "well-deserved leisure" and they want "to continue to be productive" (Rowe & Kahn, 1998). We need to clarify how much leisure is optimal to the older adult. How much is productive engagement? What balance of the two in later life leads to increased well-being?

We are in the midst of a longevity revolution. How we will spend time in these extended years is not fully determined, and the possibilities are numerous. It is to be hoped that we can be purposeful in the roles and expectations that we create for this new "third age" of human life. We need to define the possibilities and create the opportunities based on knowledge about what improves society and what improves the health, mental health, and life satisfaction of our large older population. Our 21st century society may seek the involvement of its older citizenry in work, volunteer, and caregiving roles, and the baby boomers and subsequent generations may seek increased involvement. How we shape and support these roles and how we match opportunity to capacity and preference may influence the impact of these activities on older adults as well as on their families and communities.

ENDNOTES

1. Engagement in the labor market is reflected by labor force participation rates, which measure the people in the labor force (working or actively seeking work) as a percentage of the noninstitutionalized population 15 years old and over (Kaufman & Hotchkiss, 2003).

2. Many factors may explain the variance in current levels of volunteering engagement. Volunteering is defined differently, and timing of the survey may reflect seasonal or temporary volunteering differences. Inclusion of volunteer organization types affects the findings; for example, the American Volunteer Study in 1965 excluded political and religious activities (Chamber, 1993).

3. FMLA applies to all employers meeting the following criteria: (1) public agencies, and (2) private-sector employers who employed 50 or more employees in 20 or more work weeks in the current or preceding calendar year and who are engaged in commerce or in any industry or activity affecting commerce. To be eligible for benefits, an employee must have (1) worked for a covered employer, (2) worked for the employer for a total of 12 months, (3) worked at least 1,250 hours over the previous 12 months, and (4) work at a location in the United States or in any territory or possession of the United States where at least 50 employees are employed by the employer within 75 miles.

4. "Cash and Counseling" are demonstration programs through which low-income dependent elders receive public money and education/advice to make their own care arrangements, including paying relatives to provide care.

REFERENCES

Abraham, I. L., Arrington, D. T., & Wasserbauer, L.I. (1996). Using elderly volunteers to care for the elderly: Opportunities for nursing. *Nursing Economics, 14*(4), 232-238.

Abt Associates Inc. (2001). *A profile of AmeriCorps members at baseline.* Report prepared for Corporation for National Community Service. Retrieved December 22, 2002, from http://www.americorps.org/research/pdf/servicestudy.pdf.

Administration on Aging. (n.d.). *National family caregiver support program.* Retrieved Jan 15, 2003, from http://www.aoa.gov/carenetwork/NFCSP-description.html.

Aguirre International. (2001a). *Senior companions: Accomplish report.* Report prepared for the Corporation for Community and National Service. Retrieved August 15, 2002, from http://www.seniorcorps.org/research/pdf/SCPfinal.pdf.

Aguirre International. (2001b). *RSVP: Accomplishment report.* Report prepared for the Corporation for Community and National Service. Retrieved August 15, 2002, from http://www.seniorcorps.org/research/pdf/RSVPfinal.pdf.

American Association of Retired Persons. (2001). *The policy book: AARP public policies 2001.* Washington, DC: AARP.

Aquino, J. A., Russell, D. W., Cutrona, C. E., & Altmaier, E. M. (1996). Employment status, social support, and life satisfaction among the elderly. *Journal of American Psychology, 43*(4), 480–489.

Bass, S. A., & Caro, F. G. (2001). Productive aging: A conceptual framework. In N. Morrow-Howell, J., Hinterlong, & M. Sherraden (Eds.), *Productive aging: Concepts and challenges* (pp. 37–80). Baltimore: Johns Hopkins University.

Bass, S.A., Caro, F.G., & Chen, Y. (Eds.). (1993). *Achieving a productive aging society.* Westport, CT: Auburn House.

Bass, S. A., Quinn, J. F., & Burkhauser, R. V. (1995). Toward pro-work policies and programs for older Americans. In S. Bass (Ed.), *Older and active: How Americans over 55 are contributing to society* (pp. 263–294). New Haven: Yale University.

Berkman, L. F., & Breslow, L. (1983). *Health and ways of living: The Alameda County study.* New York: Oxford University Press.

Bull, M. (1990). Factors influencing family caregiver burden and health. *Western Journal of Nursing Research, 12,* 758–776.

Bureau of Labor Statistics. (2002). *Volunteering in the United States.* Retrieved January 9, 2003, from http://www.bls.gov/news.release.volun.nr0.htm.

Bureau of Labor Statistics. (2003). *Labor force (Demographic) data.* Retrieved January, 2003, ftp://ftp.bls.gov/pub/special.requests/ep/labor.force/clfa8000.txt.

Burkhauser, R., & Quinn, J. (1997). *Implementing pro-work policies for older Americans in the twenty-first century.* Paper prepared for the United States Senate Subcommittee on Aging Forum on Older Workers. Retrieved January 2003, from http://ideas.repec.org/p/boc/bocoec/378.html

Butler, R.N. (1997). Living longer, contributing longer. *The Journal of the American Medical Association, 278*(16), 1372–1374.

Cantor, M.H. (1983). Strain among caregivers: A study of experience in the United States. *The Gerontologist, 23,* 597–604.

Carden, M. (2001). *Service learning and older adults.* St. Louis: Center for Social Development, Washington University.

Caro, F. G., & Bass, S. A. (1992). *Patterns of productivity among older Americans.* Boston: Gerontology Institute, University of Massachusetts Boston.

Caro, F. G., & Bass, S. A. (1995). Increasing volunteering among older people. In S. A. Bass (Ed.), *Older and active: How Americans over 55 are contributing to society* (pp. 71–96). New Haven, CT: Yale University.

Caro, F. G., & Morris, R. (2003). Devolution and aging policy: Introduction to the Special Issue on Devolution. *Journal of Aging and Social Policy, 14*(3/4).

Center for Disease Control. (1999). United States life tables. *National Vital Statistics Report, 47,* 28.

Center for Human Resources. (1999). *Summary report: National evaluation of Learn and Serve America.* Brandis University.

Chamber, S. M. (1987). *Good deeds in old age: Volunteering by the new leisure class.* Lexington, MA: Lexington Books.

Chambre, S. M. (1984). Is volunteering a substitute for role loss in old age? An empirical test of activity theory. *The Gerontologist, 24*(3), 292–298.

Chambre, S. M. (1993). Volunteerism by elders: Past trends and future prospects. *The Gerontologist, 33*(2), 221–228.

Chao, E., & Fiala, G. (2001). *The Older American Act Amendments of 2000: Legislative changes to the Senior Community Service Employment Program.* U.S. Department of Labor and Office of Policy and Research. Retrieved September 2002, from http://wdr.doleta.gov/opr/fulltext/01-scsep.pdf.

Cnaan, R. A., & Cascio, T. A. (1999). Performance and commitment: Issues in management of volunteers in human service organizations. *Journal of Social Service Research, 24*(3/4), 1–37.

Commission on Family and Medical Leave. (1996). *A workable balance: Report to congress on family and medical leave policies.* Retrieved January 15, 2003, from http://www.dol.gov/esa/regs/compliance/whd/fmla/firstpa.pdf.

Conner, K. A., Dorfman, L. T., & Thompkins, J. B. (1985). Life satisfaction of retired professors: The contribution of work, health, income, and length of retirement. *Educational Gerontology, 11*(4–6), 337–347.

Dautzenberg, M. G. H., Diederiks, J. P. M., Philipsen, H., & Tan, F. E. S. (1999). Multigenerational caregiving and well-being: Distress of middle-aged daughters providing assistance to elderly parents. *Women and Health, 29*(4), 57–74.

Doty, P. (1995). Older caregivers and the future of informal caregiving. In S. Bass (Ed.), *Older and active: How Americans over 55 are contributing to society* (pp. 97–121). New York: Yale University.

Earned Income Credit (EIC). (2003). Publication 596. Cat. No. 15173A. Department of the Treasury, Internal Revenue Service.

Ekerdt, D. (1986). The busy ethic: Moral continuity between work and retirement. *The Gerontologist, 26*(3), 239–244.

Ekerdt, D. (1995). Retirement. In George Maddox (Ed.), *The encyclopedia of aging* (pp. 819–823). New York: Springer Publishing Co.

Esterling, B., Kiecolt-Glaser, J., Bodnar, J., & Glaser, R. (1994). Chronic stress, social support, and persistent alterations in the natural killer cell response to cytokines in older adults. *Health Psychology, 13*(4), 291–298.

Everard, K.M., Lach, H.W., Fisher, E.B., & Baum, M.C. (2000). Relationship of activity and social support to the functional health of older adults. *The Gerontologist, 55B*(4), S208–S212.

Faison, K. J., Faria, D. H., & Frank, D. (1999). Caregivers of chronically ill elderly: Perceived burden. *Journal of Community Health Nursing, 16*(4), 243–253.

Fengler, A. P. (1984). Life satisfaction of subpopulations of elderly: The comparative effects of volunteerism, employment, and meal site participation. *Research on Aging, 6*(2), 189–212.

Fisher, B., Day, M., & Collier, C. (1998). Successful aging: Volunteerism and generativity in later life. In D. Redburn & R. McNamara (Eds.), *Social gerontology* (pp. 43–54). Westport: Auburn.

Fisher, L. R., & Schaffer, K. B. (1993). *Older volunteers: A guide to research and practice.* Newbury Park: Sage.

Foster, L., Brown, R., Carlson, B., Phillips, B., & Schore, J. (2000). *Cash and counseling: Consumer's early experiences in Arkansas:, Executive Summary.* Report prepared for U.S. Department of Health and Human Services.

Freedman, M. (1994). *Seniors in national and community service: A report prepared for the Commonwealth Fund's Americans over 55 at work program.* Philadelphia: Public/Private Ventures.

Freedman, M. (1999). *Prime time: How baby boomers will revolutionize retirement and transform America.* New York: Perseus Books/Public Affairs.

Freedman, M. (2001). Structural lead: Building the new institutions for an aging America. In N. Morrow-Howell, J. Hinterlong, & M. Sherraden (Eds.), *Perspectives on productive aging: Concepts and challenge* (pp. 245–259). Baltimore: Johns Hopkins University.

Freedman, M. (2002). *Making policy for an aging century: Expanding the contribution of older Americans through national and community service.* Warrenton, VA: Coming of Age Conference 2002.

Gallagher, S. K. (1994). Doing their share: Comparing patterns of help given by older and younger adults. *Journal of Marriage and the Family, 56,* 567–578.

Gallo, W. T., Bradley, E. H., Siegal, M., & Kasl, S. V. (2000). Health effects of involuntary job loss among older workers: Findings from the health and retirement survey. *Journal of Gerontology, 55B*(3), S131–S140.

Gary, B., & Quinn, J. (2000, January 26–27). *Retirement trends and policies to encourage work among older Americans.* Paper prepared for the annual conference of the National Academy of Social Insurance, Washington, DC.

George, L. K., & Gwyther, L. P. (1986). Caregiver well-being: A multidimensional examination of family caregivers of demanded adults. *The Gerontologist, 26*(3), 253–259.

Gonyea, J. (1997). The real meaning of balancing work and family. *The Public Policy and Aging Report, 8,* 1–8.

Goode, W. J. (1960). A theory of role strain. *American Sociological Review, 25*(4), 483–496.

Grana, J. M., & Yamashiro, S. M. (1987). *An Evaluation of the Veterans Administration Housebound and Aid and Attendance Allowance Program: Executive Summary.* Report prepared for U.S. Department of Health and Human Services.

Herz, D., & Philip, L. (1989). Institutional barriers to employment of older workers. *Monthly Labor Review, 12*(4), 14–21.

Herzog, A. R., & Morgan, J. N. (1993). Formal volunteer work among older Americans. In S. A. Bass, F. G. Caro, & Y. Chen (Eds.), *Achieving a productive aging society* (pp. 119–142). Westport: Auburn.

Herzog, A. R., House, J. S., & Morgan, J. N. (1991). Relation of work and retirement to health and well-being. *Psychology and Aging, 6*(2), 202–211.

Herzog, A. R., Kahn, R.L., Morgan, J. N., Jackson, J. S., & Antonucci, T. C. (1989). Age difference in productive activities. *Journal of Gerontology, 44*(4), S129–S138.

Hill, E. (2002, September). The labor force participation of older women: Retired? Working? Both? *Monthly Labor Review, 125*(9), 39–48.

Hinterlong, J. E. (2002). *Productive engagement and well-being in later life: A study of activity types, levels, and patterns.* Unpublished doctoral dissertation, Washington University, St. Louis.

Hooyman, N. R., & Gonyea, J. (1995). *Feminist perspectives on family care: Policies for gender justice.* Thousand Oaks, CA: Sage.

House, J. S., Landis, K. R., & Umberson, D. (1988). Social relationships and health. *American Assn. for the Advancement of Science, 241*(4865), 540–545.

Hunter, K. I., & Linn, M. W. (1980–1981). Psychological differences between elderly volunteers and non-volunteers. *International Journal of Aging and Human Development, 12*(3), 205–213.

Independent Sector. (2002). *America's senior volunteers.* Retrieved December 22, 2002, from http://www.indepsec.org/programs/research/senior_volunteers_in_america.html.

Internal Revenue Service. (2001). *Publication 503: Child and dependent care expenses*. Washington, DC: Department of the Treasury.

Intrieri, R. C., & Rapp, S. R. (1994). Self-control skillfulness and caregiver burden among help-seeking elders. *Journal of Gerontology, 49*(1), P19–P23.

Kasl, S. V., & Jones, B. A. (2000). The impact of job loss and retirement on health. In L. F. Berkman & I. Kawachi (Eds.), *Social epidemiology* (pp. 118–136). New York: Oxford University Press.

Kaufman, B. E., & Hotchkiss, J. L. (2003). *The economics of labor market* (6th ed.). Mason, OH: Thomson.

Kaye, L. W., & Alexander, L. (1995). Perceptions of job discrimination among lower-income, elderly part-timers. *Journal of Gerontological Social Work, 23*(3–4), 99–120.

Kim, J. (2003). Working paper for the Center for Social Development, Washington University.

Kollmann, G. (2000). *Social security: summary of major changes in the Cash Benefit Program*. Retrieved September 2002, from http://www.law.cornell.edu/socsec/spring01/readings/crs_history_2000.htm

Kramer, B. J. (1997). Caregiving as a life course transition among older husbands: A prospective study. *The Gerontologist, 39*(6), 658–667.

Lechner, V. M., & Gupta, C. (1996). Employed caregivers: A four-year follow-up. *Journal of Applied Gerontology, 15*(1), 102–115.

Linsk, N. L., Keigher, S. M., Simon-Rusinowitz, L., & England, S. E. (1992). *Wages for caring: Compensation family care of the elderly*. New York: Praeger.

Litigation Support Services. (1984). *Impact evaluation of the Foster Grandparent Program on the foster grandparents*. Washington, DC: ACTIOM.

Marks, N. F. (1998). Does it hurt to care? Caregiving, work-family conflict, and midlife well-being. *Journal of Marriage and the Family, 60*, 951–966.

Mathers, C. D., & Schofield, D. (1998). The health consequences of unemployment: The evidence. *Medical Journal of Australia, 168*(4), 178–182.

Moen, P., Dempster-McClain, D., & Williams, R. M., Jr. (1989). Social integration and longevity: An event history analysis of women's roles and resilience. *American Sociological Review, 54*, 635–647.

Moen, P., Dempster-McClain, D., & Williams, R. W. Jr. (1992). Successful aging: A life course perspective on women's multiple roles and health. *American Journal of Sociology, 97*(6), 1612–1638.

Moen, P., Robinson, J., & Dempster-McClain, D. (1995). Caregiving and women's well-being: A life course approach. *Journal of Health and Social Behavior, 36*, 259–273

Mor-Barak, M. E., & Wilson, S. (in press). Labor force participation of older adults: Benefits, barriers, and social work interventions. In L. Kay (Ed.), *Perspectives on productive aging: Social work with the new aged*. New York: NASW.

Mor-Barak, M. E. (1995). The meaning of work for older adults seeking employment: The generativity factor. *Internal Journal of Aging & Human Development, 41*(4), 325–344.

Mor-Barak, M. E., Scharlach, A. E., Birba, L, & Sokolov, J. (1992). Employment, social network, and health in the retirement years. *Internal Journal of Aging & Human Development, 35*(2), 145–159.

Morris, R., & Caro, F. (1996). Productive retirement: Stimulating greater volunteers efforts to meet national needs. *The Journal of Volunteer Administration, 14*(2), 5–13.

Morrow-Howell, N., Hinterlong, J., Rozario, P., & Tang, F. (2003). The effects of volunteering on the well-being of older adults. *Journal of Gerontology, 53B*(3), S137–S145.

Morrow-Howell, N., Carden, M., & Sherraden, M. (in press). Productive engagement of older adults: Volunteerism and service.

Morrow-Howell, N., Hinterlong, J., Sherraden, M., & Rozario, P. (2001). Advancing research on productivity in later life. In N. Morrow-Howell, J., Hinterlong, & M. Sherraden (Eds.), *Productive aging: Concepts and challenges* (pp. 285–311). Baltimore: Johns Hopkins University.

Muscik, M. A., Herzog, A. R., House, J. S. (1999). Volunteering and mortality among older adults: Findings from a national sample. *Journal of Gerontology: Social Science, 54B*(3), S173–S180.

Neal, M. B., Ingersoll-Dayton, B., & Starrels, M. E. (1997). Gender and relationship differences in caregiving patterns and consequences among employed caregivers. *The Gerontologist, 37*(6), 804–816.

Nightingale, D. (1998). *Implications and opportunities in the Workforce Investment Act for the Senior Community Service Employment Program.* Urban Institute. Retrieved October 2002, from http://www.urban.org/welfare/scsep.html

Noonan, A. E., & Tennstedt, S. L. (1997). Meaning in caregiving and its contribution to caregiver well-being. *The Gerontologist, 37*(6), 785–794.

Okun, M. A. (1993). Predictors of volunteer status in a retirement community. *International Journal of Aging and Human Development, 36*(1), 57–74.

Peace Corps. (2002a). *Fast facts.* Retrieved December 24, 2002, from http://www.peacecorps.gov/about/facts.cfm.

Peace Corps. (2002b). *Fast facts.* Retrieved December 24, 2002, from http://www.peacecorps.gov/benefits/financial.cfm.

Peace Corps. (n.d.). *History: The 1960s.* Retrieved December 24, 2002, from http://www.peacecorps.gov/about/history/decades/60s.cfm.

Peter D. Hart Research Associates. (1999). *The new face of retirement: Older Americans, civic engagement, and the longevity revolution.* New York: Peter D, Hart Research Associates.

Purcell, P. (2000). Older workers: Employment and retirement trends. *Monthly Labor Review, 123*(100), 19–20.

Riley, M. W., Kahn, R. L., & Foner, A. (Eds.). (1994). *Age and structural lag:*

Societies' failure to provide meaningful opportunities in work, family, and leisure. New York: John Wiley & Sons.

Robinson, K. (1990). Predictors of burden among wife caregivers. *Scholarly Inquiry for Nursing Practice, 4,* 189–208.

Rowe, J. W., & Kahn, R. L. (1998). *Successful aging.* New York: Pantheon.

Rozario, P. A. (2000). *Policy implications of family caregiving of frail elderly: Structuring the private spheres.* Area Specialization Statement. St. Louis: George Warren Brown School of Social Work, Washington University.

Rushing, B., Ritter, C., & Burton, R. P. D. (1992). Race differences in the effects of multiple roles on health: Longitudinal evidence from a national sample of older men. *Journal of Health and Social Behavior, 33*(2), 126–139.

Samorodov, A. (1999). Aging and Labor Market for Older Workers. Employment and Training Papers. Geneva: International Labor Office.

Scharlach, A. E. (1994). Caregiving and employment: Competing or complimentary roles? *The Gerontologist, 34*(3), 378–385.

Schulz, R., & Beach, S. R. (1999). Caregivng as a risk factor for mortality: The caregiver health effects study. *The Journal of the American Medical Association, 282*(3), 2215–2219. (online available: www.jama.org).

Schulz, R., O'Brien, A., Bookwala, J., & Fleissner, K. (1995). Psychiatric and physical morbidity effects of Alzheimer's disease caregiving: Prevalence, correlates, and causes. *Gerontologist, 35*(6), 771–791.

Schulz, R., Visintainer, P., & Williamson, G. M. (1990). Psychiatric and physical morbidity effects of caregiving. *Journal of Gerontology, 45*(5), P181–P191.

Seltzer, M. M., & Li, L. W. (2000). The dynamics of caregiving: Transitions during a three-year prospective study. *The Gerontologist, 40*(2), 165–178.

Senior Citizen's Freedom to Work Act of 2000. P.L.106-182. 114 Stat. 198. National Archive and Records Administration. Retrieved October 2002, from http://www.access.gpo.gov/nara/publaw/106publ.html

Senior Corps. (2002a). *Senior corps resources.* Retrieved December 23, 2002, from http://www.seniorcorps.org/resources/income_guidelines.html.

Senior Corps. (2002b). *Research: Senior companion program review.* Retrieved December 23, 2002, from http://www.seniorcorps.org/research/overview_scp01.html.

Senior Corps. (2002c). *Research: Foster grandparents program review.* Retrieved December 23, 2002, from http://www.seniorcorps.org/research/overview_fgp01.html.

Senior Corps. (2002d). *Research: RSVP overview.* Retrieved December 24, 2002, from http://www.seniorcorps.org/research/overview_rsvp01.html.

Service Leader. (1999). *Advice for volunteers: Tax credits for volunteering costs.* Retrieved December 24, 2002, from http://www.serviceleader.org/advice/taxes.html.

Shelton, A. (2000). *The Social Security earnings limit and work and retirement incentives.* Publication ID: DD54. Washington, DC: AARP.

Sherraden, M., Morrow-Howell, N., Hinterlong, J., & Rozario, P. (2001). Productive aging: Theoretical choices and directions. In N. Morrow-Howell, J., Hinterlong, & M. Sherraden (Eds.), *Productive aging: Concepts and challenges* (pp. 260–284). Baltimore: John Hopkins University.

Smith, D.H. (1994). Determinants of voluntary association participation and volunteering: A literature review. *Nonprofit and Voluntary Sector Quarterly, 23*(3), 243–263.

Spitze, G., Logan, J. R., Joseph, G., & Lee, E. (1994). Middle generation roles and the well-being of men and women. *Journal of Gerontology, 49*(3), S107–S116.

SRA Technologies. (1985). Senior Companion program impact evaluation. Washington, DC: ACTION.

Stone, R. I., & Keigher, S. M. (1994). Toward an equitable, universal caregiver policy: The potential of financial supports for family caregivers. *Journal of Aging and Social Policy, 6*(1/2), 57–75.

Strawbridge, W. J., Wallhagen, M. I., Shema, S. J., & Kaplan, G. A. (1997). New burdens or more of the same? Comparing grandparents, spouse, and adult child caregivers. *The Gerontologist, 37*(4), 505–510.

Sundeen, R. A. (1992). Difference in personal goals and attitudes among volunteers. *Nonprofit and Voluntary Sector Quarterly, 21*(3), 271–291.

Tennstedt, S., Cafferata, G. L., & Sullivan, L. (1992). Depression among caregivers of impaired elders. *Journal of Aging & Health, 4*(1), 58–76.

Tennstedt, S. (1999, March). *Family caregiving in an aging society.* Paper presented at the Administration on Aging's Symposium on Longevity in the New Century.

The Catalog of Federal Domestic Assistance. (n.d.). *59.026 Service Corps of Retired Executives Association.* Retrieved December 20, 2002, from http://www.cfda.gov/static.p59026.htm.

Thoits, P. A., & Hewitt, L. N. (2001). Volunteer work and well-being. *Journal of Health and Social Behavior, 42*(2), 115–131.

Townsend, A., Noelker, L., Deimling, G., & Bass, D. (1989). Longitudinal impact of interhousehold caregiving on adults children's mental health. *Psychology and Aging, 4*(4), 393–401.

U.S. Department of Health and Human Services. (2002). *HHS Approves Expanded "Independent Choices" in Arkansas.* HSS news, released on October 2, 2002.

U.S. Department of Veterans Affairs. (n.d.). *Self-evaluation to promote community living for people with disabilities.* Report prepared for the President on Executive Order 13217.

U.S. Bureau of Census. (1996). *Statistical abstract of the United States: 2001.* Washington, DC: U.S. Government Printing Office.

U.S. Bureau of Census. (2001). *Statistical abstract of the United States: 2001.* Washington, DC: U.S. Government Printing Office.

U.S. Equal Employment Opportunity Commission. (1997). *The Americans with Disabilities Act of 1990.* P.L. 101-336. Retrieved October 2002, from http://www.eeoc.gov/laws/ada.html

U.S. General Accounting Office. (2001). *Older workers: Demographic trends pose challenges for employers and workers.* Report to the Ranking Minority Member, Subcommittee on Employer-Employee Relations, Committee on Education and the Workforce, House of Representatives. Washington, DC: U.S. Government Printing Office.

U.S. House and Representatives. U.S. Committee on Ways and Means. (2000). *Green Book. Section 1: Social Security: The Old-Age, Survivors, and Disability Insurance (OASDI) Program.* Washington, DC: U.S. Government Printing Office.

Uccello, C. (1998). *Factors influencing retirement: Their implications for raising retirement age.* Urban Institute. Retrieved October 2002, from http://www.urban.org/socsecurity/retire_factors.pdf

USA Freedom Corps. (2002). *USA Freedom Corps: Principles and reforms for a citizen service act.* Retrieved December 22, 2002, from http://www.whitehouse.gov/infocus/communityservice/book.pdf.

Van Willigen, M. (2000). Differential benefits of volunteers across the life course. *Journal of Gerontology, 55B*(5), S308–S318.

Vitaliano, P., Scanlan, J., Krenz, C., & Fujimoto, W. (1996a/b). Insulin and glucose: Relationships with hassles, anger and hostility in nondiabetic older adults. *Psychosomatic Medicine, 58*(5), 489–499.

Wagner, D. L. (1997). *Comparative analysis of caregiver data for caregivers to the elderly 1987 and 1997.* Report for National Alliance for Caregiving.

Walker, A. J., Shin, H., & Bird, D. N. (1990). Perceptions of relationship change and caregiver satisfaction. *Family Relations: Journal of Applied Family & Child Studies, 39*(2), 147–152.

Wallsten, S. S. (2000). Effects of caregiving, gender, and race on the health, mutuality and social supports of older couples. *Journal of Aging and Health, 12*(1), 90–111.

Warburton, J., Brocque, R., & Rosenman, L. (1998). Older people—the reserve army of volunteers? An analysis of volunteerism among older Australians. *International Journal of Aging and Human Development, 46*(3), 229–245.

Westat. (1998). *Effective practices of foster grandparents in Head Start Center.* Report prepared for Corporation for National Service. Retrieved December 23, 2002, from http://www.seniorcorps.org/research/pdf/fgp_hs.pdf.

White-Means, S. I., & Thornton, M. C. (1996). Ethnic differences in the production of informal home health care. *The Gerontologist, 30*(6), 758–768.

Wilcox, S., & King, A.C. (1999). Sleep complaints in older women who are family caregivers. *Journal of Gerontology, 54B*(3), P189–P198.

Wilson, J. (2000). Volunteering. *Annual Review of Sociology, 26,* 216–240.

Yee, J. L., & Schulz, R. (2000). Gender differences in psychiatric morbidity among family caregivers: A review and analysis. *The Gerontologist, 40*(2), 147–164.

Zarit, S. H., Gaugler, J. E., & Jarrott, S. E. (1999). Useful services for families: Research findings and directions. *International Journal of Geriatric Psychiatry, 14*(3), 165–181.

CHAPTER 3

From Successful Aging to Conscious Aging

Harry R. Moody

> A human being would certainly not grow to be seventy or eighty years
> old if this longevity had no meaning for the species. The afternoon
> of human life must also have a significance of its own and cannot be
> merely a pitiful appendage to life's morning.
>
> —Carl Jung

When we look at our globe from a planetary perspective we recognize that population growth is slowing and that populations are aging. United Nations demographers estimate that by the middle of this current century global population will peak and then begin to decline, a process chiefly attributable to rapid decreases in fertility in both the industrialized and the developing world. Does this leveling of population mean the decline of humanity? On the contrary, it means an achievement of equilibrium, ecologically speaking, and the opening of a new chapter in the human story (Mumford, 1956). What does this new chapter entail? Specifically, what does a new planetary ecological balance involve in psychological or symbolic terms, in terms of how we think of ourselves and of the human future?

Within two decades, Americans over 65 years of age, instead of being one in eight (as of now) in the population, will be one in five—a dramatically larger proportion. In the nations of Japan and

Western Europe, this shift is already further advanced. Developing countries will move in this direction as well. What will this shift mean for the economy, for family life, for the health care system? For those who unconsciously identify growth with sheer size or quantitative expansion, population aging provokes unease, even gloom (Moody, 1988). An aging population represents a shadow across the face of things to come and, psychologically speaking, it represents the shadow part or the unexamined dimension of our future selves.

As a storm at sea approaches land, signs in the sky are evident before the storm reaches the shore. So, too, there are signs that this enormous transformation of population aging is already having its effect on our understanding of ourselves and on our image of the second half of life.

The Face of Aging. The face of aging in America is changing. We are moving away from a negative image (the "ill-derly") toward a more positive image (the "well-derly"). The current sea change is prompted by rising longevity and health, by an exploding population of aging baby boomers, and by emerging deals of growth and development over the life span. A survey of periodical literature over the 20th century confirms this shift away from managing problems of aging in favor of health promotion and contributions toward the well-being of society (Holkup, 2001). This development is one chapter in an older story of ambivalence about aging, which historian Thomas Cole called "bipolar ageism" (Cole, 1992). We vacillate between hope and fear, between negative stereotypes of old age and positive elixirs that promise the secret of overcoming time and aging itself (McHugh, 2003).

The current shift can be summarized, in slogan form at least, by two phrases that redefine a shared understanding of what aging might mean:

- the first is **Successful Aging** (sometimes called "Vital Aging" or "Active Aging")
- the second is **Productive Aging** (often linked to "redefining retirement")

Successful Aging is the expectation that later life can be a time of sustained health and vitality. Successful aging appeals to individual hopes and dreams: "You should live and be well." Productive aging is the expectation that later life should be a time not for disengagement but for a continued contribution to society, through worklife extension, volunteerism, or other contributive roles. Both ideals—sometimes subsumed under the label of "The New Gerontology"—amount to a new, more positive version of later life: rejection of familiar notions of old age as a social problem in favor of the idea of aging as an opportunity for the individual and society (Rowe, 1997; Gergen and Gergen, 2001). Both successful aging and productive aging represent the attraction of gerontology by the power of positive thinking, a hardy perennial in American life. But these deeply rooted cultural ideals of growth and expansion also may represent a refusal to face the "shadow" side of aging itself (Zweig and Abrams, 1991).

Successful Aging: Science or Ideology? In this chapter, I want to look critically at the new positive image of aging—not so much to reject it, as some commentators have done (Holstein & Minkler, 2003), but to understand what social and psychological conditions are required if the ideals are ever to become more than a slogan. Specifically, I want to look at the shadow elements neglected by our embrace of the new gerontology. I have elsewhere described successful aging and productive aging as different elements of an ideology: that is, a system of ideas that expresses, and simultaneously conceals, underlying human interests (Moody, 2001). To grasp this point about ideology, it is enough to note that in the United States, anything that appeals to success and productivity is likely to prove decisive, because values of success and productivity are so deeply embedded in the national character.

Where does the agenda of successful aging come from? How will it evolve in the future? First, note that the notion of successful aging is not exactly a new idea. The hope that later life could be a period of vitality and activity was first expressed in Cicero's treatise, *De Senectute*. The outlines of Cicero's view are parallel to what Rowe and Kahn (1998) would develop in their book, *Successful Aging*. Apparently, it took the MacArthur Successful Aging project millions of dollars to discover what a Roman philosopher stumbled upon 2,000 years ago and expressed so eloquently in his classic treatise.

But, in all fairness, the MacArthur Foundation was not mistaken to undertake its project. The MacArthur researchers needed to justify their conclusions by science, not by philosophical speculation. That fact makes all the difference in terms of the credibility of successful aging for Americans today. To be persuasive, an ideology must be accepted as true, not merely useful, to human interests of different kinds. Proponents of successful aging want us to believe it is not mere opinion, still less an ideology (as I have suggested). Indeed, in the spirit of positivism, successful aging is presented as *a fact*, the way things are, in contrast to old-fashioned prejudice (i.e., ageism). This rhetorical foundation for successful aging is based on rejecting myths: for example, the mistaken idea that the course of later life is foreordained by fate or genetic determinism. To the contrary, Rowe and Kahn reassure us, if only we open our mind to the facts, we will see that our condition in old age is largely up to us.

Now, it would be unfair to criticize Successful Aging simply as Horatio Alger in geriatric dress. But we do have to recognize an unmistakable appeal here to personal autonomy and individual responsibility ("A healthy old age is up to you!"), which is certainly a message Americans will respond to.

This characteristically American cultural approach to successful aging demands that we look more carefully at Rowe and Kahn's original formulation of the idea. They distinguish *successful* aging from *normal* aging. Following their formulation, subsequent debate about successful aging has tended to assume that success in coping with aging means delaying the features of normal aging. Thus, for someone gifted with successful aging, to be 80 years old means looking and acting like a 70 year old, and so on. But, as Torres (1999) points out, this prevailing understanding of successful aging enshrines an activity- and future-oriented set of values. "Managing on one's own becomes prized above all else. Refusal of dependency is understandable insofar as dependency in caregiving often leads to loss of dignity (Lustbader, 1991). But the result of uncritically accepting the prevailing version of successful aging is that "dignity" becomes equated with independence, thus reitifying individualist values and neglecting cross-cultural variations in patterns of family caregiving. Not all situations of caregiving entail loss of dignity.

What is needed to correct this misunderstanding is both more refined empirical work and a more thoughtful critique of the atheoretical patterns of social gerontology, which has long been a problem in the field. For example, some recent empirical work in Sweden by Torres and colleagues has involved looking more closely at the relationship between cultural values and successful aging: specifically, at value orientations around relational modes and social networks (Torres, 1999). Whether dependency entails loss of dignity will be heavily influenced by such cultural differences, not be physical traits alone. In short, different cultures, even today, view self-sufficiency in ways that are profoundly different.

What is clear is that taking for granted our individualist, activity-oriented, and future-oriented approach to successful aging becomes an uncritical kind of cultural blindness (a kind of ethnocentrism) that will not be overcome by empirical investigation by itself. Empiricism alone will not correct the problem. Offering more precise correlations between locus of control and life-satisfaction and then extrapolating these findings to ideas about autonomy or successful aging simply disregards the cultural context in which people live their lives. A genuinely critical gerontologist would attempt to bring such presuppositions to the surface, and Holstein and Minkler's critique is in the spirit of critical gerontology (Minkler & Estes, 1999).

Varieties of Successful Aging. A comprehensive review of the term successful aging in the academic literature turned up a variety of definitions. But different uses of the term converge on key ideas such as life satisfaction, longevity, freedom from disability, mastery and growth, active engagement with life, and independence. The preponderant emphasis here is on maintaining positive functioning as long as possible (Phelan & Larson, 2002). Against this progress-oriented version of successful aging, this review also acknowledged a certain fluidity tied to a diversity of socioeconomic variables. Thus, individual progress is balanced by tolerance and relativism in characteristically American fashion.

By contrast, British gerontologist Alan Walker avoids the term successful aging in favor of *active* aging, which he links to five policy domains: employment, pensions, retirement, health, and citizenship (Walker, 2002). Focusing mainly on Europe, Walker believes that a policy strategy on behalf of active aging can be justified on both an ethical basis (greater equality) and an economic basis (reduced old age dependency). In contrast to American proponents of successful aging, Walker's approach focuses on population and the life course: that is, he looks beyond individualism and emphasizes long-range consequences of habits of early life (Bower, 2001). When we look at the new gerontology from a global, international perspective, it becomes clear why analysts in other countries outside the United States prefer the concept of active aging instead of successful aging. The semantic difference suggests a deeper divergence between images of positive aging in America in contrast to the rest of the world (World Health Organization, 2002). Again, the ethnocentrism of the dominant version of successful aging is apparent.

Finally, let us note that even critics of Rowe and Kahn's approach—for instance, those who favor a religious or spiritual view—seem to accept the premise that successful aging represents happy and healthy aging. For example, Crowther and her colleagues (2002) have argued that spirituality is a forgotten factor in the successful-aging paradigm. But they end up arguing that spirituality or religiosity (the two are often conflated) is a factor that promotes better physical and mental health in old age. This line of argument—"Religion is good for your health" will certainly have its appeal (Koenig, 1999). But it amounts to accepting all too quickly the basic premise of Rowe and Kahn's initial formulation of successful aging.

The Power of Positive Thinking. Before we too quickly dismiss Rowe and Kahn's formulation, we need, again, to look carefully at their text. When we do look closely, we note that the book actually contains not one, but two different definitions of successful aging. The first definition, the one discussed up to this point, is couched in terms of maximum wellness: avoidance of disease and disability and active engagement with life. A good old age, in this definition, is just an old age with minimum sickness or frailty, as much like youth or midlife as possible.

On this point, Rowe and Kahn bring forward the idea of "compression of morbidity" (Fries & Crapo, 1995) originally articulated by Oliver Wendell Holmes in his poem "The Wonderful One-Horse Shay," which is cited in their book. Compression of morbidity is not exactly "prolongevity," but it is a descendent of the same progressivist spirit (Gruman, 2003). We can think of compression of morbidity as a bit like political liberalism, in contrast to revolutionary political ideology. Political liberalism works within the system to promote progress without challenging limits. By contrast, revolutionary ideology wants to overthrow the status quo. So too, compression of morbidity doesn't promise we will live longer than the maximum life span in previous epochs, but incremental progress is still assured.

Compression of morbidity, and successful aging, are mainstream, liberal ideologies, whereas appeals to so-called anti-aging medicine are revolutionary and reject the dogmas of mainstream biology and medicine. Even if their present claims are bogus, this goal of "uncapping" maximum life span may not be impossible. However, these prospects lie outside what Rowe and Kahn understand successful aging to be. Their liberal incremental version of successful aging means that, as far we can, we postpone sickness (morbidity) until the very end of life and then die quickly, without lingering illness or debility. This is a hopeful, but realistic, version of progress in successful aging, couched in terms of individual responsibility and initiative: the triumph of contemporary American values.

Decrement with Compensation. Now, interestingly enough, a close reading of Rowe and Kahn's book turns up a quite different definition of Successful Aging, a definition expressed by the phrase "decrement with compensation." Like compression of morbidity, decrement with compensation is easy enough to understand. In this case, the goal of positive aging is not to stay healthy longer and longer but, rather, to adapt, to make the best of our situation, even if it means chronic illness and decline. Instead of postponing decline, we recognize that decline is to be expected, and so we compensate for it and adapt to it.

Successful aging, in this second version, does not mean remaining healthy as long as possible but adapting to losses when they occur. For example, instead of downhill skiing, one takes up cross-country skiing. Instead of remaining a professional athlete, one becomes a coach; and so on. This definition of successful aging is more realistic in acknowledging the limits of individual autonomy. No matter how vigorous one's efforts at health promotion, anyone can succumb to accidents and the failings of advanced age. In statistical terms there is steady increase of chronic illness and frailty in later life and Gompertz's law (first formulated in 1828) still confirms that the rate of mortality in human beings doubles every 8 years.

Successful Aging, then, comes in to two quite different versions. The first version stakes the whole meaning of success on avoiding bad outcomes and preserving health and vitality as long as possible. The second version looks for compensating factors and invites us to ask just what sorts of compensation might be possible, either individually or societally. I will come back to this point later, but for now it is enough to see that the two definitions of successful aging are very different in their implications. Curiously, they are never quite reconciled by Rowe and Kahn. Most commentators, especially those who attack the idea of successful aging, have concentrated their fire entirely on the first definition while ignoring the second.

The ideal of successful aging— understood in its first version as indefinite prolongation of the values of middle-age—is a prescription for remaining on a superficial level of life: "Hold on to what you've got as long as possible." By contrast, when losses demand a new approach—the second definition of successful aging as "decrement with compensation"—we have the potential for going beyond, or below, that superficial level of life. Once we take seriously the second version of successful aging, then, age itself can be an opportunity for spiritual growth, as in the Sufi saying "When the heart grieves for what it has lost, the spirit rejoices for what it has found." It is this spiritual opportunity—what we may call "conscious aging"—that I turn to now.

Meeting the Shadow. Drew Leder (Leder, 2000) accurately pinpoints the attractiveness of successful aging in terms of a Western model of combating losses as best as we can. He contrasts this with what he terms "spiritual aging," that involves embracing losses as a curriculum for developing the soul: "Age challenges us to see beyond the ego-self, now falling into disrepair. Who am I, if not just this wrinkled face in the mirror?" The advent of illness in later life sometimes proves to be the trigger for this call, or "descent into the underworld," which is an encounter with a deeper level of living, as psychiatrist Jean Shinoda Bolen describes it:

> When life is lived superficially or is almost entirely outer-directed, something has to happen that leads to soul-searching. Until then, there may be very little communication between the upperworld and the underworld, between the inner world of the personal and collective unconscious and the outer-world concerns of the ego. Layers of facade, of entitlement, and privilege that were built up over the years have no bearing on the occurrence or progression of an illness, and do not adequately prepare a person for the underworld descent. (Bolen, 1998, p. 70)

If we can no longer sustain the midlife values of maximum wellness and productivity, then the descent will trigger troublesome questions not asked earlier in life:

> Illness raises questions: Who are you when you stop doing? When you cannot be productive or are no longer indispensable to others? When you can no longer go on as before because you are sick, when you lose status? Who are you when you can't be a caretaker or a boss or do your job, whatever this might be? Do you matter?

If we listen to these questions—those posed in the second version of successful aging as decrement with compensation—then we move along a different path from the prolongation of the values held supreme in the first half of life:

> The truth that will set us free in the last half of our lives is not to be found in ego complexification. Consciousness has a developmental quality in the first half. In our old age, it grows through disenvelopment. It moves backward. It is a regression in the service of transcendence (Bouklas, p. 300).

Bouklas writes from his long experience as a geriatric psychotherapist. Yet his conclusions echo our second version of successful aging. True, decrement with compensation rings like the jargon of abstract social science and the phrase "regression in the service of transcendence" does little to improve it. Yet, these ideas reflect a profound truth that the greatest artists have conveyed in their lives and works.

Late Freedom. Take the case of Beethoven, who experienced an ultimate narcissistic wound with sensory disability that attacked the very core of his creative identity. In his Heiligenstadt testimony, Beethoven recorded his own descent into despair and soul-searching (Sullivan, 1960). After he became totally deaf, he went on to produce the Ninth Symphony. His last years were a creative journey rooted in the solitude of inner silence. One could imagine a Beethoven who never lost his hearing but went on to produce more and more symphonic creations that pushed the limits of classical form, just as the first version of successful aging would simply prolong the virtues of midlife. But Beethoven was forced to take the path of descent and solitude. He produced the ninth symphony and the late string quartets, and he burst the limits of conventional form in the service of musical transcendence (Solomon, 2003).

Beethoven did not live into old age, but this pattern of creative response to disability—decrement with compensation—is recognized in other great artists. Some artists—Picasso is a great example—demonstrate the first version of successful aging: productive engagement, activity, and prolongation of the values of youth and midlife (Schiff, 1984). But others are forced to undergo descent and decrement.

One of the most brilliant examples is the late work of Matisse, produced when the old artist suffered physical infirmities that confined him to a wheelchair and prevented him from painting large canvasses. Instead, Matisse turned to cutting out colored pieces of cardboard. These cut-outs represented a radical simplification of his lifelong style (Elderfield, 1978). In keeping with the continuity theory of aging, Matisse never lost his passionate love of color. But in his later years, the evocation of color became simplified, purified, and transformed into that late freedom seen in so many artists in old age (Dormandy, 2000). Matisse demonstrated not ego complexification but a sublime kind of regression, a simplicity that was the fruit of a lifetime's experience.

The Virtues of Age. So we may wonder: Is the dominant version of successful aging an expression of our wider antiaging culture? In his critique of the contemporary ideology of successful aging, Stephen Katz (2001) points to the ascendance of ideas grouped under categories such as postmodernism and posthumanism. Katz notes that the appeal of timelessness and self-reliance is tied to the promise of technology and the mirage of overcoming all limits. As a marketing agenda, successful aging tends to blend imperceptibly into antiaging (Katz, 2001). From cosmetic surgery to lifelong learning, from virtual bodies to the prosthetic self, the appeal is always to turn away from outdated images of maturity in favor of a reinvented identity outside of time and finitude. By contrast, Katz urges us to reflect more deeply about the true resources of temporality—the resources of tradition, wisdom, narrative, memory, and generativity—that affirm intrinsic values of aging instead of dwelling exclusively on risk and loss (Katz & Marshall, 2003).

Let us push this matter of risk and loss to its ultimate extreme and ask the question: Is it possible to find successful aging in a nursing home? If we adopt the first version of it (prolonged wellness), then evidently not. But what about the second version, decrement with compensation? Here it is appropriate to point out that Erik Erikson, modern-day prophet of the virtues of the life cycle, died in a nursing home, as did his wife Joan. We have no testimony about their final days in a long-term care facility and can only speculate about it. But we do have a remarkable record of successful aging in a nursing home: The journal of Florida Scott-Maxwell (Berman, 1986). Her powerful words give a new meaning to the idea of decrement with compensation:

> Another secret we carry is that though drab outside—wreckage to
> the eye, mirrors a mortification— inside we flame with a wild life that

is almost incommunicable . . . It is a place of fierce energy. Perhaps passion would be a better word than energy, for the sad fact is that this vivid life cannot be used. If I try to transpose it into action, I am soon spent. It has to be accepted as passionate life, perhaps the life I never lived, never guessed I had it in me to live. It feels other and more than that. It feels like the far side of precept and aim. It is just life, the natural intensity of life, and when old, we have it for our reward and undoing. (Scott-Maxwell, 1968, pp. 32–33)

Rarely have we heard words that so vividly convey the dialectical truth of losses balanced by gains, physical decline compensated by spiritual insight. The message of Florida Scott-Maxwell's nursing home journal is not far from the spirit of Rembrandt's late self-portraits, the visual record of a long journey toward ego-integrity achieved in the midst of losses and tragedy. What Rembrandt's late-life portraits convey are the same qualities some psychologists have discerned in successful aging: self-acceptance, inner mastery, purpose in life, and personal growth (Ryff, 1989).

The testimony of great artists converges with life-span developmental theories and clinical concepts of personal growth. Whether in Matisses's cutouts, in Florida Scott-Maxwell's nursing home journal, or Rembrandt's self-portraits, we find the same recurring motif. Personal meaning is sustained through inner resources permitting continued growth even in the face of loss, pain, and physical decline. This compensation for decrement arises from a spiritual core that makes transcendence a genuine path in the last stage of life (Moody, 2002). The inspiring account by Ram Dass of his struggle with a near-fatal stroke evokes the same message, the same decrement with compensation, that we have seen repeatedly in those who have made the descent and returned (Ram Dass, 2001).

Shared Transcendence. Is this gero-transcendence limited to great artists or writers (Tornstam, 1997)? Not at all. Collings (2001) conducted an empirical study of successful aging among the Inuit people on Victoria Island in the Canadian Archipelago. It turned out that the Inuit people understand elderhood in much the same way as our own society. But they do not share the first version of successful aging (active engagement and good health). Instead, successful old age was viewed as the ability to manage declines in health in a positive way. The key element was understood as a capacity to transmit accumulated wisdom to the next generation. Rabello de Castro and Rabello de Castro's case studies (2001) of Brazilian elders came to a similar conclusion: coping mechanisms of successful aging reflect ways in which we constitute a sense of meaning in terms of a total life history, not gains or losses at a particular point in time.

This entire line of ethnographic research underscores the way in which successful aging—understood as decrement with compensation—depends in crucial ways on what Bourdieu would call *social capital*, especially the cultural and symbolic resources that provide a sense of meaning when the mask of midlife achievement slips away (Marin, 2001). Even in the American environment, we know that social networks and social relationships are of enormous importance for sustaining cognitive function associated with successful aging (Seeman et al., 2001). In contrast to the individualism (a la Horatio Alger) of the first version of successful aging, these sources of compensation are correlated with the social capital and the resources of the wider society. Instead of looking to elders on the ski slopes, we need to look at elders in wheelchairs who can inspire us with examples of successful aging in the face of chronic illness (Poon et al., 2003).

With this wider perspective—society's instead of the individual's—we come, full circle, to the question with which I began this exploration: namely, how do we come to see human aging in the widest ecological, planetary perspective? The prophets of gloom see in population aging only a loss because they have not listened to the testimony of those who have gone through the descent and returned with a message of hope. Coming full circle means coming to recognize the circle of life, which is compensation for finitude and a glimpse of what lies beyond. As the Celtic proverb puts it; "Make time a circle, not a line." When we regain this vision, a vision of the great circle of life, successful aging becomes conscious aging.

REFERENCES

Berman, H. J. (1986). To flame with a wild life: Florida Scott-Maxwell's experience of old age. *Gerontologist, 26*(3), 321–324.

Bolen, J. S. (1998). *Close to the bone: Life-threatening illness and the search for meaning.* New York: Scribner.

Bouklas, G. (1997). *Psychotherapy with the elderly: Becoming Methuselah's echo.* Lantham, MD: Jason Aronson.

Bower, B. (2001). Healthy aging may depend on past habits. *Science News, 159*(24), 373.

Cole, T. (1992). *The journey of life: A cultural history of aging in America.* New York: Cambridge University Press.

Collings, P. (2001). "If you got everything, it's good enough": Perspectives on successful aging in a Canadian Inuit community. *Journal of Cross-Cultural Gerontology, 16*(2), 127–155.

Crowther, M. R., Parker, M. W., Achenbaum, W. A., Larimore, Walter L., & Koenig, H. G. (2002, October). Rowe and Kahn's Model of Successful Aging revisited: Positive spirituality—The forgotten factor. *Gerontologist, 42*(5), 613–620.

Dormandy, T. (2000). *Old masters: Great artists in old age.* London: Hambledon Press.

Elderfield, J. (1978). *The cut-outs of Henri Matisse.* New York: George Braziller.

Fries, J. F., & Crapo, L. M. (1995). *Vitality and aging: Implications of the rectangular curve.* New York: W.H. Freeman.

Gergen, M. M., & Gergen, K. J. (2001–2002, Winter). Positive aging: New images for a new age. *Ageing International, 27*(1), 3–23.

Gruman, G. J. (2003). *A history of ideas about the prolongation of life: The evolution of prolongevity hypotheses to 1800.* New York: Springer Publishing.

Holkup, P. A. (2001, June). 20th Century. *Journal of Gerontological Nursing, 27*(6), 38–46.

Holstein, M., & Minkler, M. (2003, December). Self, society and the new gerontology. *Gerontologist, 43*(6), 787–796.

Katz, S. (2001–2002, Winter). Growing older without aging? Positive aging, anti-ageism, and anti-aging. *Generations, 25*(4), 27–32.

Katz, S., & Marshall, B. (2003, February). New sex for old: Lifestyle, consumerism, and the ethics of aging well. *Journal of Aging Studies, 17*(1), 3–16.

Kimble, M. A., & McFadden, S. H. (Eds.). (2003). *Aging, spirituality, and religion: A handbook* (Vol. 2, pp. 422–433). Minneapolis, MN: Fortress Press.

Koenig, H. G. (1999). *The healing power of faith.* New York: Simon & Schuster

Leder, D. (2000). The trouble with successful aging. Retrieved from http://www.secondjourney.org/reprint_series/leder1/leder1_p1.htm

Lustbader, W. (1991). *Counting on kindness: The dilemmas of dependency.* New York: Free Press.

McHugh, K. E. (2003, March). Three faces of ageism: Society, image and place. *Ageing and Society, 23*(2), 165–185

Marin, M. (2001). Successful ageing—Dependent on cultural and social capital? Reflections from Finland. *Indian Journal of Gerontology, 15*(1–2), 145–159.

McHugh, K. E. (2003, March). Three faces of ageism: Society, image and place. *Ageing and Society, 23,* 165–185.

Minkler, M., & Estes, C. (1999). *Critical gerontology: Perspectives from political and moral economy.* Amityville, NY: Baywood.

Moody, H. (1988). *Abundance of life: Human development policies for an aging society.* New York: Columbia University Press.

Moody, H. (2002). Conscious aging: The future of religion in later life. In M. A. Kimble & S. H. McFadden (Eds.), *Handbook of religion, spirituality and aging* (2nd ed., pp. 422–433). Minneapolis: Fortress Press.

Moody, H. (2001). Productive aging and the ideology of old age. In N. Morrow-Howell (Ed.), *Perspectives on productive aging* (pp. 175–196). Baltimore: Johns Hopkins University Press.

Morrow-Howell, N., Hinterlong, J., & Sherraden, M. W. (Eds.). (2001). *Productive aging: Concepts and challenges* (pp. 175–196). Baltimore: Johns Hopkins University Press.

Mumford, L. (1956). *Transformations of man.* New York: Harper and Row.

Phelan, E. A., & Larson, E. B. (2002, July). Successful aging—Where next? *Journal of the American Geriatrics Society, 50*(7), 1306–1308.

Poon, L. W., Gueldner, S. H., & Sprouse, B. M. (Eds.). (2003). *Successful aging and adaptation with chronic diseases.* New York: Springer Publishing.

Rabello de Castro, L., & Rabello de Castro, G. (2001). Coping in old age: Considerations from the point of view of case studies from Brazil. *Indian Journal of Gerontology, 15*(1–2), 181–197.

Ram Dass. (2001). *Still here: Embracing aging, changing, dying.* New York: Riverhead Books.

Rowe, J. W. (1997). The new gerontology. *Science, 278,* 367.

Rowe, J., & Kahn, R. (1998). *Successful aging.* New York: Random House.

Ryff, C. D. (1989, March). Beyond Ponce de Leon and life satisfaction: New directions in quest of successful ageing. *International Journal of Behavioral Development, 12*(1), 35–55.

Schiff, G. (1984). *Picasso: The last years, 1963–1973.* New York: George Braziller.

Scott-Maxwell, F. (1968). *The measure of my days.* New York: Penguin.

Seeman, T. E., Lusignolo, T. M., Albert, M., & Berkman, L. (2001). Social relationships, social support, and patterns of cognitive aging in healthy, high-functioning older adults: MacArthur studies of successful aging. *Health Psychology, 20*(4), 243–255.

Solomon, M. (2003). *Late Beethoven: Music, thought, imagination.* Los Angeles: University of California Press.

Sullivan, J. W. N. (1960). *Beethoven: His spiritual development.* New York: Random House.

Tornstam, L. (1997, Summer). Gerotranscendence: The contemplative dimension of aging. *Journal of Aging Studies, 11*(2), 143–154.

Torres, S. (1999). A culturally-relevant theoretical framework for the study of successful ageing. *Ageing and Society, 19*(1), 33–51.

Walker, A. (2002, January–March). Strategy for active ageing. *International Social Security Review, 55*(1), 121–139.

World Health Organization. (2002). *Active ageing: A policy framework.* Geneva, Switzerland: World Health Organization.

Zweig, C., & Abrams, J. (1991). *Meeting the shadow: The hidden power of the dark side of human nature.* Los Angeles: Jeremy Tarcher.

PART II

What Constitutes Successful Aging?

Diana L. Morris

T he first chapter in this section deals with the beneficial effects of exercise for the elders, while the second focuses on the importance of maintaining a health diet. Both diet and exercise help the aging process, promote health and have been shown to halt physical deterioration and often improve bodily functioning. In the third chapter, the authors describe a model of successful aging that is applied to elders who are impacted by the effects of chronic illness. The section addresses ways that elders can take care of themselves to avoid or reduce the negative effects of aging.

The first chapter by Roberts and Adler examines the health effects of exercise for elders. Although many neglect to exercise regularly, it is known that exercise activities can provide many beneficial effects, such as improved cardiovascular functioning, muscle strength, balance, minimization of existing physical impairments, and promote mental health. On the other hand, health problems can arise and intensify without the benefit of regular exercise. The authors assert that it is ideal for older adults to exercise with partners, and emphasize intergenerational exercise in families, where support and encouragement is readily available. Identified in the chapter are three types of exercise: aerobic, muscle strength-training, and flexibility or range of motion activities, each providing respective physical benefits. Though exercise is seen as a burden by many, as long as it is approached with safety in mind in a supportive atmosphere, it promotes a more healthy future for aging persons.

Dietary patterns and their effects on successful aging are the focus of the second chapter. Although food consumption patterns are widely taken for granted, they remain one of the most important factors for health aging. Much progress has recently been made in researching diet patterns and needs throughout life's stages, showing that poor diet can be associated in the leading causes of death in the United States, including cancer, stroke, heart disease, and Alzheimer's disease. Dietary components, such as caloric intake, protein, calcium, and a range of vitamins, all function when properly managed to guard against adverse health conditions. The author states that as aging progresses, diets inevitably change as body processes slow and energy levels decrease. As one ages, the result is lower caloric requirements making it more difficult for elders to maintain optimal levels of nutrient consumption. The take home message is that despite the widely varying personal dietary requirements needed to remain healthy, moderation is best for successful aging.

The third chapter by Kahana aims to remove the negative connotations associated with chronically ill elders who cannot participate fully in the practices of successful aging. The author outlines a model for successful aging and then applies that model to the circumstances of elders who are chronically ill. Preventive Adaptations are described that include health promotion, planning ahead, and helping others. Corrective Adaptations encompass marshalling support, role substitution, and engaging in activity and environmental modifications. Emergent Adaptations refers to technology use, health care consumerism, and self-improvement. The Kahana chapter proceeds to apply the three models of adaptation to four chronic health conditions: arthritis, heart disease, diabetes, and cognitive impairment. Next is an illustration of three individual cases and how each elder incorporates components of successful aging while chronically ill. The chapter reiterates that typically the solutions and problems of the aging process are complex and highly specific for each individual, yet a proactive approach to aging despite the presence of chronic illness can still lead to success in aging.

CHAPTER 4

Exercise and the Generations

Beverly L. Roberts and Patricia A. Adler

T he health effects of exercise are well-known, and increasing the exercise in persons of all ages is a major national goal described in Healthy People 2010 (United States et al., 2000). In spite of the benefits of exercise, many do not engage in regular exercise at intensities high enough to achieve beneficial effects. Models of behavior change have provided some understanding of the mechanisms leading to the incorporation of regular exercise into daily activities. Those persons who have a partner to exercise with are more likely to maintain an exercise program. However, the influence of intergenerational partners has been largely ignored. These partners may increase adherence to exercise and demonstrate the importance of it to persons of all ages. This chapter explores some of the health benefits of exercise among elderly adults. Topics include exercise prescription, the role of intergenerational exercise groups in beginning, and maintaining a regular exercise program.

EXERCISE AND HEALTH

With advancing age, impairments in motor tasks increased difficulty in performing daily activities (Roberts, 1999). These impairments are often the result of chronic disease, aging and a sedentary lifestyle. To a certain extent, exercise can reverse the effects of these factors but cannot take the place of appropriate management of chronic disease or irreversible age related physical changes. Research regarding exercise is voluminous, and no attempt will be made to summarize it. However, the effects of exercise on motor tasks and activities of daily living will be examined because of their importance to the independence of elderly adults.

Nagi's model of the mechanisms contributing to disability (Nagi, 1991) will be used to organize the literature on effects of exercise on the health of older adults because of its simplicity, explanatory power and relevance to independence in daily activities. In this model, pathology leads to functional impairments that are disruptions in physiologic systems or anatomical structure. These impairments lead to functional limitations that are physical, cognitive, and psychological, and they contribute to disability—that is, difficulty in performing socially acceptable roles. The functional impairments selected for this review are those that contribute to motor tasks required for daily activity and include aerobic capacity, muscle strength, and balance. Also, the functional limitations selected for this review are gait and activity intolerance. Activities of daily living are the subject of this review because of their importance to the independence of older adults. Depression also will be examined because it is an intraindividual factor that contributes to functional limitations and disability (Pope & Tarlov A, 1991; Verbrugge & Jette, 1994).

Functional Impairment

The benefits of aerobic exercise on cardiovascular function are well established and include, for example, lower blood pressure, increased stroke volume, and lower resting heart rate. Several types of aerobic exercise have produced significant increases in cardiovascular function and aerobic capacity. While aerobic capacity increased with endurance training of only one muscle group (Tyni-Lenne, Gordon, Jansson, Bermann, & Sylven, 1997), changes were significantly greater, as muscle mass used in the exercises also increased (Harrington et al., 1997a). Hence, exercise that involves more of the large muscle groups will have a greater effect than exercise only using a few or small muscle groups. Examples of aerobic exercise that use very large muscle groups are walking, running, swimming, and biking.

Aerobic exercise also significantly increases muscle strength and balance, which are requisites for safe walking and transferring and for independence in daily activities. Impaired muscle function, muscle atrophy, and decreased muscle strength contribute to progressive disability (Coats et al., 1992).

Muscle strength is a requisite for ambulation, moving from lying, sitting, and standing positions and performing activities of daily living. The strength of muscles in the lower extremity is essential to performing these motor tasks. In independent functionally mobile adults aged 62 to 88 years, seven muscle groups in the lower body accounted for 14% to 31% of variance in the time to negotiate an obstacle course that required motor tasks also needed for daily activities. Moreover, the importance of muscle strength increased as the tasks became more difficult (Lamoureux, Sparrow, Murphy, & Newton, 2002).

Exercise has other beneficial effects on muscles. Aerobic exercise was associated with peripheral changes in the ability of muscles to generate energy and to activate muscle fibers more efficiently (Adamopoulos et al., 1993; Afzal, Brawner, & Keteyian, 1998; Harrington & Coats, 1997a; McKelvie et al., 1995; Ohtsubo et al., 1997a; Stratton et al., 1994a). Hence, not only is strength increased, but also muscle contraction and muscle coordination become more efficient.

Tasks requiring a greater proportion of muscle strength also are perceived to be more challenging. Older adults with lower reserves in strength may perceive even common tasks, such as climbing stairs, as being difficult and avoid these activities (Pescatello & Judge, 1995). Even essential daily tasks can be a problem for persons who have poor muscle strength. Thus, muscle strengthening programs have the potential to increase the activities that older adults engage in because they may perceive the activities as less difficult.

Balance is dependent on muscle strength, particularly of the lower extremities (Lord, Clark, & Webster, 1991; Roberts, Wagner, Palmer, Mansour, & Srour, 1993; Tideiksaar, 1995). Among elderly adults, an 8-week aerobic walking program increased balance (Roberts, 1989). Similar findings were found with a 12-week aerobic walking program (Roberts, Srour, Mansour, Palmer, & Wagner, 1994), one year aerobic exercise program (Lord, Ward, & Williams, 1996b) and a one year program of walking, cycling and jogging (Brown & Holloszy, 1993). Other types of aerobic exercise programs had similar outcomes (Ferrucci et al., 2000; Lord, Ward, & Williams, 1996a; Lord, Ward, Williams, & Strudwick, 1995; Roberts, 1989).

Functional Limitations

Muscle strength and balance are integral to gait, which is essential for mobility. During a 3-year period, the onset of the inability to walk was related to decreases in strength and balance (Rantanen

et al., 2001). Balance is required for safe ambulation and performance of daily activities. Balance was positively associated with gait
and getting up from a chair (Ferrucci et al., 2000; Lord et al., 1996;
Rantanen et al., 1998; Rantanen & Avela, 1997) and was predictive
of subsequent disability (Guralnik, Ferrucci, Simonsick, Salive, &
Wallace, 1995). Although poor gait was related to difficulty in transferring and toileting (Simonsick et al., 2001), it also adversely
affects the performance of such activities as heavy housework, shopping, and light housework.

Even in very old and frail older adults, muscle strengthening
programs significantly improve motor tasks such as gait. A 3-week
program of aerobic exercise increased the distance walked (Meyer
et al., 1997b). A 12-week aerobic walking program improved gait
(Roberts, Srour, Woollacott, & Tang, 1994). Mechanisms for
changes in gait may be related to greater motor control (Friedman,
Rickmond, & Basket, 1988), decreased energy needed for gait
(Meyer et al., 1997b) and improved balance and muscle strength
(Roberts, 1999).

Gait is essential to motor tasks related to activities of daily living.
In contrast, activity tolerance is related to the duration that an older
adult can perform the task without fatigue or excessive shortness of
breadth. Aerobic exercise, in particular, has been associated with
increases in activity tolerance. One of the mechanisms for the
increase in activity tolerance is the consistent finding that aerobic
exercise improves aerobic capacity, which refers to the capacity for
metabolism of oxygen to produce the energy required for daily
activities. Several types of aerobic exercise have produced significant increases in cardiovascular function, aerobic capacity, and
exercise tolerance (Belardinelli, Georgiou, Cianci, & Purcaro, 1999;
Belardinelli, Georgiou, Scocco, Barstow, & Purcaro, 1995; Hambrecht et al., 1995; Harrington et al., 1997b; Keteyian et al., 1996;
Kiilavuori, Sovijarvi, Naveri, Ikonen, & Leinonen, 1996; Meyer et al.,
1996; Shephard, Kavanagh, & Mertens, 1998). Although the effects
of exercise on exercise tolerance and aerobic capacity were thought
to be primarily related to central cardiovascular function, the
peripheral changes in the ability of muscles to generate energy and
to activate muscle fibers more efficiently are equally important in
explaining the mechanisms by which exercise increases activity
tolerance (Adamopoulos et al., 1993; Afzal et al., 1998; Harrington
& Coats, 1997b; McKelvie et al., 1995; Ohtsubo et al., 1997b; Stratton et al., 1994b). Although increased muscle strength has been

associated with increases in activity tolerance (Mancini et al., 1992), the effects of muscle strengthening exercise programs on activity intolerance have not been well established.

Disability

Difficulty in performing ADLs has primarily been the focus of nearly 30 years of geriatric research that primarily has focused on functional impairments (muscle strength and balance) and functional limitations (gait and basic motor tasks such as getting up from a chair). Little attention has been given to the modifications that allow people to complete the activities or to the exertion associated with them. People make accommodations to be able to perform daily activities (e.g., rest periods, assistive devices) (Roberts, 1999), hence, may be able to perform these activities but not efficiently or with great effort. Activities requiring a great amount of exertion or modification to be completed may be done less often, or not at all (Roberts, 1999). The role of exercise in disability is not clear because there are few studies of the effects of exercise on activities of daily living. In small studies, aerobic exercise increased independence in daily activities (Coats, Adamopoulos, Meyer, Conway, & Sleight, 1990; Greenland & Chu, 1988; Gulanick, 1991), and a muscle strengthening program increased the ability to perform daily activities (Duncan et al., 1998; Mihalko & McAuley, 1996). In contrast, others did not find that exercise significantly reduced restriction in daily activities (Meyer et al., 1997a).

EXERCISE PRESCRIPTION

The selection of an exercise program begins with an exercise prescription comprised of type of exercise (aerobic, resistance, range of motion), frequency, and duration. Safety is an essential consideration for any exercise program. A health check is advised if there is any question about the appropriateness of the individual to participate in exercise.

Types of Exercise

There are three types of exercise, and each offers different benefits for health. Aerobic exercise involves repetitive movements of the large muscle groups, and improves cardiovascular, respiratory and musculoskeletal function; it also decreases blood pressure, improves mood, increases high-density lipoproteins, and inhibits osteoporosis (Tratora & Grabowski, 1993). Muscle strength-training involves movement against resistance, which increases the strength of muscles, tendons, and ligaments; promotes joint stability; and improves circulation to the joint and surrounding tissues (Lam, 2003). Flexibility or range of motion exercise, such as yoga, involves active movement of the joints that increases joint flexibility by gently stretching and strengthening the adjoining soft tissue of the joint (Lam, 2003).

Selection of an exercise can begin with taking into consideration physical activities that participants perform every day. For elders and those in poor physical condition, walking is done with nearly every activity and is a safe and familiar exercise that does not require learning a new motor behavior, such as riding a bike. Walking is adaptable to all weather conditions because it can be done outside or inside in places such as a mall or store. For example, participants can walk while shopping for groceries. Elderly adults with joint problems and decreased endurance may have less difficulty, and feel safer, using a shopping cart for support while walking. Walking can also be combined with pleasurable activities such as going to the movies while parking the car so persons need to walk a little further.

Frequency, Intensity, and Duration

The American College of Sports Medicine (1995) recommends exercise of 30 minutes three times a week. More frequent exercise with moderate duration is recommended for older adults (American College of Sports Medicine, 1995). The recommended intensity of exercise is generally less for older adults than for younger adults and children. A general guideline is that exercise is at the correct intensity when the participant can carry on a comfortable conversation. Depending on the person's response to exercise, the duration of exercise may also need to be gradually increased from short (10–20 minutes) to longer periods (20–45 minutes). To prevent injury, warm-up and cool-down exercises should be included in any exercise program and should consist of stretching and low intensity exercise such as walking at a normal pace.

Special Considerations for Older Adults

The best advice for safe exercise is to engage in exercise that does not exacerbate a preexisting condition. One key to success is to begin slowly and gradually increase the duration of exercise. Elderly adults tolerate low to moderate exercise best, which a younger person may perceive as being of very low intensity (American College of Sports Medicine, 1995). Chronic age-related conditions, such as arthritis, obesity, and heart disease prevent many older adults from engaging in high intensity exercise intensity (e.g., running, skiing, and hiking) that may also significantly increase the risk of injury or death during exercise. To avoid injury, older adults, in particular, should avoid the impulse to push themselves beyond their limits and through pain. Older adults must know when to stop exercise (e.g., when excessive fatigue, extreme weakness, or chest pain occurs) and reassess either the suitability of the exercise or its duration or intensity.

Fear of falling is a real concern of older adults, particularly if they fell in the past during exercise (Bruce, Devine, & Prince, 2002). However, the fear of falling may not be consistent with physical and environmental factors that may contribute to the risk of falls (Roberts, 1999). The health care provider can assess physical abilities and help the older adult select an exercise that can be done safely. Moreover, an exercise leader also can modify the exercise to be consistent with the older adult's physical abilities. However, any exercise leader must understand the effects of aging and treatment of chronic illnesses on the ability to exercise safely. The book, *Exercise: A Guide from the National Institute on Aging,* is a very good resource for older adults, and the accompanying video can be used to guide the exercise session.

Despite the recognized benefits of exercise in elders, the development of effective strategies to encourage their exercise participation remains a challenge. Long-term adherence to an exercise program is the desired outcome of an appropriate and effective exercise prescription. Factors that influence adherence to a fitness program in elders include confidence of the person or self-efficacy (Allison & Keller, 2000; Brassington, Atienza, Perczek, DiLorenzo, & King, 2002; Conn, 1998), social support (Rhodes et al., 2000; Rhodes et al., 1999), physical frailty (Rhodes et al., 1999), and barriers to the accessibility and availability of exercise (Jones & Jones,

1997). That successful engagement in exercise is important because it builds confidence in the older person's ability and readiness to maintain an exercise program.

Many exercise programs in various venues such as senior centers and the YMCA promote exercise in older adults, including individual and group exercise programs utilizing home, hospital, and community settings. The social support provided by group programs increases participation and adherence to regular exercise (Gillett, 1988). Follow-up contact with participants also improves exercise adherence (Castro, King, & Brassington, 2001; Sullivan, Allegrante, Peterson, Kovar, & MacKenzie, 1998).

As noted by Moore (1996), the current cohort of older women comes from an age when women were not expected to exercise, and they may need more encouragement and may prefer low intensity exercise. Older men, on the other hand, often recall pleasant memories about participation in sports in their adolescent and young adult years. Thus, older men may be more likely to be attracted to exercise similar to that in their younger years.

INTERGENERATIONAL EXERCISE

Intergenerational exercise provides an opportunity for persons from all generations to engage in a fun activity that bolsters the relationship among participants. Having fun together also means growing together with a sense of social connection. The challenge of intergenerational exercise is to find an exercise that all participants can engage in safely.

Exercise should be safe and age appropriate and, perhaps more important, elders and young children should feel safe. Although some older adults may be more physically active than their younger family members and could serve as role models in promoting exercise, preexercise assessments by a health care provider may be needed. Older persons usually are at risk for injury because of concomitant cardiac disease and may require a stress test before starting an exercise program (American College of Sports Medicine, 1995). Family members with other chronic conditions such as arthritis, hypertension, or pulmonary disease should consider activity limitations that may have been prescribed when planning an exercise program. It is important that persons of all ages do not feel compelled to engage in exercise beyond their personal comfort or physical abilities.

To insure the safety and fun for all, consistency in the prescriptions for all members of all ages who will be exercising together must be taken into consideration. The types and duration of exercise may be very diverse, especially when the very young or old are included. Although older adults and the very young can participate in other exercise such as bicycle riding, care must be taken to take into consideration the physical abilities, past experience with exercise, and deconditioning when planning an intergenerational program. Tai Chi, yoga, and walking are low intensity exercise and are good options when family members include the very old and the very young. The challenge of participants of intergenerational exercise is to identify an exercise program that accommodates the needs of all participating generations while insuring that all can enjoy the activity.

The best advice in selecting an intergenerational exercise is to keep the plan simple and flexible so that the experience is enjoyable and safe for all. Family members should approach the subject of exercise as an opportunity for fitness and family fun that has a variety of options. Part of the fun is engaging in the decision-making process and anticipating the fun and benefits of exercise. Participants should discuss their preferences and explore exercise options. The key is to find an exercise that all family members can do and enjoy together. Equipment and exercise areas should be easily accessible to all participants.

Health care providers can offer suggestions for an exercise plan and where to find exercise programs in the community. Information about exercise programs can be found in newsletters, local newspapers, or on the Web. Senior centers and indoor shopping malls are two popular community resources where postings can be found. Some families may prefer to join an exercise activity designed to promote a particular cause, such as the Arthritis Foundation Walk. Videotapes and books can be used to learn an exercise program and may increase exercise adherence.

Family members can provide social support by encouraging exercise, but, more important, they can provide exercise partners. Families can be instrumental in reducing or eliminating factors associated with decreased adherence to exercise in persons of all ages. For example, perceived barriers to exercise adherence, such as transportation and access to equipment, may be easily addressed by car pooling or purchasing equipment that can be used by all participants. Ways in which families choose to create fun in their exercise experience will take on the personality of the family and how they relate to each other. Some may prefer to set goals and reward regular exercise participation and minimize competition. Other families may decide on a program with less structure and more flexibility.

CONCLUSION

In summary, the beneficial effects of exercise on health and function are well-known. Yet, most people of all ages are sedentary. Often, exercise is perceived as a burden or painful rather than fun (Conn, 1998). This view may deter many from beginning or maintaining an exercise program. The social support and fun that intergenerational exercise provides may increase the adherence to a regular exercise program. In all cases, family members who engage in intergenerational exercise become cheerleaders for each other's success and thus help ensure the present and future health of their families.

REFERENCES

Adamopoulos, S., Coats, A. J., Brunotte, F., Arnolda, L., Meyer, T., Thompson, C. H., et al. (1993). Physical training improves skeletal muscle metabolism in patients with chronic heart failure. *Journal of the American College of Cardiology, 21*(5), 1101–1106.

Afzal, A., Brawner, C. A., & Keteyian, S. J. (1998). Exercise training in heart failure. *Progress in Cardiovascular Diseases, 41*(3), 175–190.

Allison, M., & Keller, C. (1997). Physical activity in the elderly: Benefits and intervention strategies. *Nurse Practitioner, 22*(8), 53–4, 56, 58.

Allison, M. J., & Keller, C. (2000). Physical activity maintenance in elders with cardiac problems. *Geriatric Nursing, 21*(4), 200–203.

American College of Sports Medicine. (1995). *Guidelines for exercise testing and prescription.* Baltimore: Williams and Wilkins.

Belardinelli, R., Georgiou, D., Cianci, G., & Purcaro, A. (1999). Randomized, controlled trial of long-term moderate exercise training in chronic heart failure: Effects on functional capacity, quality of life, and clinical outcome. *Circulation, 99*(9), 1173–1182.

Belardinelli, R., Georgiou, D., Scocco, V., Barstow, T. J., & Purcaro, A. (1995). Low intensity exercise training in patients with chronic heart failure. *Journal of the American College of Cardiology, 26*(4), 975–982.

Brassington, G. S., Atienza, A. A., Perczek, R. E., DiLorenzo, T. M., & King, A. C. (2002). Intervention-related cognitive versus social mediators of exercise adherence in the elderly. *American Journal of Preventive Medicine, 23*(2 suppl.), 80–86.

Brown, M., & Holloszy, J. O. (1993). Effects of walking, jogging and cycling on strength, flexibility, speed and balance in 60- to 72-year olds. *Aging (Milano.), 5*(6), 427–434.

Bruce, D. G., Devine, A., & Prince, R. L. (2002). Recreational physical activity levels in healthy older women: The importance of fear of falling. *Journal of the American Geriatric Society, 50*(1), 84–89.

Castro, C. M., King, A. C., & Brassington, G. S. (2001). Telephone versus mail interventions for maintenance of physical activity in older adults. *Health Psychology, 20*(6), 438–444.

Coats, A. J., Adamopoulos, S., Meyer, T. E., Conway, J., & Sleight, P. (1990). Effects of physical training in chronic heart failure. *Lancet, 335,* 63–66.

Coats, J. S., Adamopoulos, S., Radaelli, A., McCance, A., Meyer, T. E., Bernardi, L., et al. (1992). Controlled trial of physical training in chronic heart failure. *Circulation, 85,* 2119–2131.

Conn, V. S. (1998). Older adults and exercise: Path analysis of self-efficacy related constructs. *Nursing Research, 47,* 180–189.

Duncan, P., Richards, L., Wallace, D., Stoker-Yates, J., Pohl, P., Luchies, C., et al. (1998). A randomized, controlled pilot study of a home-based exercise program for individuals with mild and moderate stroke. *Stroke, 29*(10), 2055–2060.

European Heart Failure Training Group. (1998). Experience from controlled trials of physical training in chronic heart failure. Protocol and patient factors in effectiveness in the improvement in exercise tolerance. *European Heart Journal, 19,* 466–475.

Ferrucci, L., Bandinelli, S., Benvenuti, E., Di Iorio, A., Macchi, C., Harris, T. B., et al. (2000). Subsystems contributing to the decline in ability to walk: Bridging the gap between epidemiology and geriatric practice in the InCHIANTI study. *Journal of the American Geriatrics Society, 48*(12), 1618–1625.

Fiatarone, M. A., & Evans, W. J. (1990). Exercise in the oldest old. *Topics in Geriatric Rehabilitation, 5,* 77.

Fiatarone, M. A., Marks, E. C., Ryan, N. D., Meredith, C. N., Lipsitz, L. A., & Evans, W. J. (1990). High-intensity strength training in nonagenarians. Effects on skeletal muscle. *Journal of the American Medical Association, 263*(22), 3029–3034.

Friedman, P. J., Richmond, D. E., & Basket, J. J. (1988). A prospective trial of serial gait speed as a measure of rehabilitation in the elderly. *Age & Ageing, 17*(4), 227–235.

Gillett, P. A. (1988). Self-reported factors influencing exercise adherence in overweight women. *Nursing Research, 37*(1), 25–29.

Greenland, P., & Chu, J. S. (1988). Efficacy of cardiac rehabilitation services. *Annals of Internal Medicine, 109*(8), 650–663.

Gulanick, M. (1991). Is phase 2 cardiac rehabilitation necessary for early recovery of patients with cardiac disease? A randomized, controlled study. *Heart & Lung, 20*(1), 9–15.

Guralnik, J. M., Ferrucci, L., Simonsick, E. M., Salive, M. E., & Wallace, R. B. (1995). Lower-extremity function in persons over the age of 70 years as a predictor of subsequent disability. *New England Journal of Medicine, 332*(9), 556–561.

Hambrecht, R., Niebauer, J., Fiehn, E., Kalberer, B., Offner, B., Hauer, K., et al. (1995). Physical training in patients with stable chronic heart failure: Effects on cardiorespiratory fitness and ultrastructural abnormalities of leg muscles. *Journal of the American College of Cardiology, 25*(6), 1239–1249.

Harrington, D., Clark, A. L., Chua, T. P., Anker, S. D., Poole-Wilson, P. A., & Coats, A. J. (1997a). Effect of reduced muscle bulk on the ventilatory response to exercise in chronic congestive heart failure secondary to idiopathic dilated and ischemic cardiomyopathy. *American Journal of Cardiology, 80*(1), 90–93.

Harrington, D., & Coats, A. J. (1997). Mechanisms of exercise intolerance in congestive heart failure. *Current Opinion in Cardiology, 12*(3), 224–232.

Hershberger, P. J., Robertson, K. B., & Markert, R. J. (1999). Personality and appointment—keeping adherence in cardiac rehabilitation. *Journal of Cardiopulmonary Rehabilitation, 19*(2), 106–111.

Jette, A. M., Rooks, D., Lachman, M., Lin, T. H., Levenson, C., Heislein, D., et al. (1998). Home-based resistance training: Predictors of participation and adherence. *Gerontologist, 38*(4), 412–421.

Jones, J. M., & Jones, K. D. (1997). Promoting physical activity in the senior years. *Journal of Gerontological Nursing, 23*(7), 40–48.

Kavanagh, T., Myers, M. G., Baigrie, R. S., Mertens, D. J., Sawyer, P., & Shephard, R. J. (1996). Quality of life and cardiorespiratory function in chronic heart failure: Effects of 12 months' aerobic training. *Heart, 76*(1), 42–49.

Keteyian, S. J., Levine, A. B., Brawner, C. A., Kataoka, T., Rogers, F. J., Schairer, J. R., et al. (1996). Exercise training in patients with heart failure. A randomized, controlled trial. *Annals of Internal Medicine, 124*(12), 1051–1057.

Kiilavuori, K., Sovijarvi, A., Naveri, H., Ikonen, T., & Leinonen, H. (1996). Effect of physical training on exercise capacity and gas exchange in patients with chronic heart failure. *Chest, 110*(4), 985–991.

Lam, P. (2003). Taijiquan in the treatment of arthritis. *Journal of Traditional Eastern Health and Fitness, Summer,* 36–40.

Lamoureux, E. L., Sparrow, W. A., Murphy, A., & Newton, R. U. (2002). The relationship between lower body strength and obstructed gait in community-dwelling older adults. *Journal of the American Geriatrics Society, 50*(3), 468–473.

Lord, S. R., Clark, R. D., & Webster, I. W. (1991). Postural stability and associated physiological factors in a population of aged persons. *Journal of Gerontology, 46*(3), M69–M76.

Lord, S. R., Lloyd, D. G., Nirui, M., Raymond, J., Williams, P., & Stewart, R. A. (1996). The effect of exercise on gait patterns in older women: A randomized controlled trial. *Journals of Gerontology: Biological and Medical Sciences, 51*(2), M64–M70.

Lord, S. R., Ward, J. A., & Williams, P. (1996). Exercise effect on dynamic stability in older women: A randomized controlled trial. *Archives of Physical Medicine and Rehabilitation, 77*(3), 232–236.

Lord, S. R., Ward, J. A., Williams, P., & Strudwick, M. (1995). The effect of a 12-month exercise trial on balance, strength, and falls in older women: A randomized controlled trial. *Journal of the American Geriatrics Society, 43*(11), 1198–1206.

Mancini, D. M., Walter, G., Reichek, N., Lenkinski, R., McCully, K., Mullen, J., et al. (1992). Contribution of skeletal muscle atrophy to exercise intolerance and altered muscle metabolism in heart failure. *Circulation, 85*(4), 1364–1373.

McCool, J. F., & Schneider, J. K. (1999). Home-based leg strengthening for older adults initiated through private practice. *Preventive Medicine, 28*(2), 105–110.

McKelvie, R. S., Teo, K. K., McCartney, N., Humen, D., Montague, T., & Yusuf, S. (1995). Effects of exercise training in patients with congestive heart failure: A critical review. *Journal of the American College of Cardiology, 25*(3), 789–796.

Meyer, K., Gornandt, L., Schwaibold, M., Westbrook, S., Hajric, R., Peters, K., et al. (1997a). Predictors of response to exercise training in severe chronic congestive heart failure. *American Journal of Cardiology, 80*(1), 56–60.

Meyer, K., Schwaibold, M., Westbrook, S., Beneke, R., Hajric, R., Gornandt, L., et al. (1996). Effects of short-term exercise training and activity restriction on functional capacity in patients with severe chronic congestive heart failure. *American Journal of Cardiology, 78*(9), 1017–1022.

Meyer, K., Schwaibold, M., Westbrook, S., Beneke, R., Hajric, R., Lehmann, M., et al. (1997b). Effects of exercise training and activity restriction on 6-minute walking test performance in patients with chronic heart failure. *American Heart Journal, 133*(4), 447–453.

Mihalko, S. L., & McAuley, E. (1996). Strength training effects on subjective well-being and physical function in the elderly. *Journal of Aging and Physical Activity, 4,* 68.

Moore, S. M., & Kramer, F. M. (1996). Women's and men's preferences for cardiac rehabilitation program features. *Journal of Cardiopulmonary Rehabilitation, 16*(3), 163–168.

Nagi, S. (1991). Disability concepts revisited: Implications for prevention. In A. M. Pope & A. R. Tarlov (Eds.), *Disability in America: Toward a national agenda for prevention* (pp. 304–327). Washington, DC: National Academy Press.

National Institute of Aging. (2001). *Exercise: Guide.* Washington DC: US Department of Health and Human Services. Retrieved June 10, 2004, from http://www.niapublications.org/exercisebook/ExerciseGuide-Complete.pdf.

Ohtsubo, M., Yonezawa, K., Nishijima, H., Okita, K., Hanada, A., Kohya, T., et al. (1997). Metabolic abnormality of calf skeletal muscle is improved by localised muscle training without changes in blood flow in chronic heart failure. *Heart, 78*(5), 437–443.

Pescatello, L. S., & Judge, J. O. (1995). The impact of physical activity and physical fitness on functional capacity in older adults. In B. S. Spivack (Ed.), *Evaluation and management of gait disorders* (pp. 325–339). New York: Marcel Dekker.

Piepoli, M. F., Flather, M., & Coats, A. J. S. (1998). Overview of studies of exercise training in chronic heart failure: The need for a prospective randomized multicentre European trial. *European Heart Journal, 19*(6), 830–841.

Pina, I. L. (1997). Exercise and heart failure. In G. J. Balady & I. L. Pina (Eds.), *Exercise and heart failure* (pp. 213–219). Armonk, NY: Futura Publishing.

Pine, M., Gurland, B., & Chren, M. M. (2002). Use of a cane for ambulation: Marker and mitigator of impairment in older people who report no difficulty walking. *Journal of the American Geriatrics Society, 50,* 263–268.

Pine, Z. M., Gurland, B., & Chren, M. M. (2000). Report of having slowed down: Evidence for the validity of a new way to inquire about mild disability in elders. *Journals of Gerontology: Biological and Medical Sciences, 55*(7), M378–M383.

Pope, A., & Tarlov, A. (1991). *Disability in America: Toward a national agenda for prevention.* Washington DC: National Academy Press.

Rantanen, T., & Avela, J. (1997). Leg extension power and walking speed in very old people living independently. *Journals of Gerontology Series A: Biological and Medical Sciences, 52*(4), M225–M231.

Rantanen, T., Guralnik, J. M., Ferrucci, L., Penninx, B. W., Leveille, S., Sipila, S., et al. (2001). Coimpairments as predictors of severe walking disability in older women. *Journal of the American Geriatrics Society, 49*(1), 21–27.

Rantanen, T., Guralnik, J. M., Izmirlian, G., Williamson, J. D., Simonsick, E. M., Ferrucci, L. et al. (1998). Association of muscle strength with maximum walking speed in disabled older women. *American Journal of Physical Medicine and Rehabilitation, 77*(4), 299–305.

Rhodes, E. C., Martin, A. D., Taunton, J. E., Donnelly, M., Warren, J., & Elliot, J. (2000). Effects of one year of resistance training on the relation between muscular strength and bone density in elderly women. *British Journal of Sports Medicine, 34*(1), 18–22.

Rhodes, R. E., Martin, A. D., Taunton, J. E., Rhodes, E. C., Donnelly, M., & Elliot, J. (1999). Factors associated with exercise adherence among older adults. An individual perspective. *Sports Medicine, 28*(6), 397–411.

Roberts, B. L. (1989). Effects of walking on balance among elders. *Nursing Research, 38,* 180–182.

Roberts, B. L. (1999). Activities of daily living: Factors related to independence. In A. Hinshaw, S. Feetham, & J. Shaver (Eds.), *Handbook of clinical nursing research* (pp. 561–577). New York: Sage.

Roberts, B. L., Srour, M. I., Mansour, J. M., Palmer, R. M., & Wagner, M. B. (1994). The effects of a 12-week aerobic walking program on postural stability of healthy elderly. In K. Taguchi, M. Igarashi, & S. Mori (Eds.), *Vestibular and neural front* (pp. 215–218). New York: Elsevier.

Roberts, B. L., Srour, M. I., Woollacott, M., & Tang, P. F. (1994). The effects of a 12-week aerobic walking program on gait of healthy elderly. In K. Taguchi, M. Igarashi, & S. Mori (Eds.), *Vestibular and neural front* (pp. 295–298). New York: Elsevier.

Roberts, B. L., Wagner, M., Palmer, R., Mansour, J. M., & Srour, M. I. (1993). Muscle strength and endurance among healthy elderly adults. *Physical Therapy, 73*(6), S37.

Roberts, B. L., & Wykle, M. L. (1993). Falls among institutionalized elderly: Pilot study results. *Journal of Gerontological Nursing, 19,* 13–20.

Sandin, K. J., & Smith, B. S. (1990). The measure of balance in sitting in stroke rehabilitation prognosis. *Stroke, 21*(1), 82–86.

Shephard, R. J., Kavanagh, T., & Mertens, D. J. (1998). On the prediction of physiological and psychological responses to aerobic training in patients with stable congestive heart failure. *Journal of Cardiopulmonary Rehabilitation, 18*(1), 45–51.

Simonsick, E. M., Kasper, J. D., Guralnik, J. M., Bandeen-Roche, K., Ferrucci, L., Hirsch, R., et al. (2001). Severity of upper and lower extremity functional limitation: Scale development and validation with self-report and performance-based measures of physical function. WHAS Research Group. Women's Health and Aging Study. *Journals of Gerontology Series B: Psychological Sciences and Social Sciences, 56*(1), S10–S19.

Stratton, J. R., Dunn, J. F., Adamopoulos, S., Kemp, G. J., Coats, A. J., & Rajagopalan, B. (1994). Training partially reverses skeletal muscle metabolic abnormalities during exercise in heart failure. *Journal of Applied Physiology, 76*(4), 1575–1582.

Sullivan, T., Allegrante, J. P., Peterson, M. G., Kovar, P. A., & MacKenzie, C. R. (1998). One-year follow up of patients with osteoarthritis of the knee who participated in a program of supervised fitness walking and supportive patient education. *Arthritis Care and Research, 11*(4), 228–233.

Tideiksaar, R. (1995). *Falls in older persons.* New York: Marcel Dekker.

Tratora, G. J., & Grabowski, S. R. (1993). *Principles of anatomy and physiology.* New York: Harper Collins.

Tyni-Lenne, R., Gordon, A., Jansson, E., Bermann, G., & Sylven, C. (1997). Skeletal muscle endurance training improves peripheral oxidative capacity, exercise tolerance, and health-related quality of life in women with chronic congestive heart failure secondary to either ischemic cardiomyopathy or idiopathic dilated cardiomyopathy. *American Journal of Cardiology, 80*(8), 1025–1029.

United States, Office of Disease Prevention and Health Promotion, United States, Office of Public Health and Science, United States, & Dept. of Health and Human Services (2000). *Healthy people 2010.* (Conference ed.; last modified: [2000-02-16] ed.) Washington, DC: U.S. Dept. of Health and Human Services, Office of Public Health and Science.

Verbrugge, L. M., & Jette, A. M. (1994). The disablement process. *Social Science and Medicine, 38*(1), 1–14.

CHAPTER 5

Food for Thought . . . and Good Health

Grace J. Petot

If we could give every individual the right amount of nourishment and exercise, not too little and not too much, we would have found the safest way to health.

—Hippocrates, c. 460–377 BC

S uccessful aging is dependent on genetic and lifelong behavioral and environmental factors. We cannot do much about our genetic heritage but are able to manage many of the other influences during our lifetime. Because we take food and eating very much for granted, dietary habits and food patterns are not often considered to make up a very large part of our personal environment. However, they represent some of the greatest influences on successful aging (Nicolas, Andrieu, Nourhashemi, Rolland, & Vellas, 2001; Weindruch & Sohal, 1997). Over the past 20 years, there has been greatly increased interest in understanding the relationships among diet patterns in early life and health and well-being in later life. These relationships represent one of the public health challenges we are facing today (Koplan & Fleming, 2000).

Among the 10 leading causes of death in the United States in 2000, 5 have been shown to implicate dietary behaviors as risk factors. They are heart disease, cancer, stroke, diabetes, and Alzheimer's disease (Anderson, 2002). We are learning that dietary habits throughout life have important implications for health and longevity. In this chapter, we will discuss the influences of several dietary components and food patterns on health and well-being.

NUTRITIONAL COMPONENTS OF DIETS RELATED TO THE CHRONIC DISEASES OF AGING

Energy (Calories)

Research studies on mice during the mid-20th century demonstrated that restricting calories but maintaining adequate nutrient adequacy in young and growing mice allowed them to live longer and postponed most of the chronic diseases of later life (Masoro, 2000; Weindruch & Sohal, 1997). Studies starting in 1987 and still continuing in primates are already demonstrating some of the same protective effects (Roth, 2001). They are expected to suffer less diabetes and fewer cardiovascular problems and may age more slowly. These kinds of experiments cannot be done in humans; however, it is possible to conclude that both caloric quantity and diet quality may enhance human longevity and quality of life (Casadesus, Shukin-Hale, & Joseph, 2002). Thus, it is important to learn more about how lifelong food habits can influence health and well-being in later life.

Evidence has been accumulating that Americans are eating more and are less physically active. Overweight and obesity, along with continuing reductions in energy expenditure are contributing to the incidence of cardiovascular diseases, diabetes, and, possibly, cancer. More Americans are eating foods away from home, and there is much evidence that portion sizes of many of these foods have been increasing over the years. Comparisons of food portion sizes reported in the United States Food and Drug Administration (USDA) Nationwide Food Consumption Survey in 1978 with those reported in 1998 show increases ranging from 49 to 183 calories per portion (Nielson & Popkin, 2003). Many portion sizes in the marketplace are 2-5 times larger than standard portion sizes established for nutrition labeling by the USDA and the FDA (Young & Nestle, 2003). Thus, many persons may be quite unaware that more calories are being consumed than expected. The combination of greater energy intake and reduced energy expenditure leads to excessive body weight that then becomes a risk factor for the development of chronic disease. Therefore, recommendations include lifetime control of total calories plus increased activity or energy expenditure.

Protein and calcium. For many years, dietary advice emphasized the importance of sufficient protein in our diets. It is true now that for most Americans, diets contain much more protein than is needed. However, for those persons with very low calorie consumption, it sometimes becomes difficult to provide enough protein to cover tissue maintenance and repair needs, because some of the protein may be utilized for energy. This is especially true for the frail elderly. In addition, protein and dietary calcium act synergistically to maintain bone health in the face of osteoporosis and recovery from fractures (Dawson-Hughes & Harris, 2002).

Vitamins B6, B12, and Folate. These vitamins are associated with the metabolism of amino acids. Low intakes or deficiencies of one or more of these vitamins may lead to the accumulation of homocysteine in the blood and become a risk factor or an indicator of risk for cardiovascular disease (Jacobsen, 1998). There are now indications that elevated homocysteine levels may also be a risk factor for dementia and Alzheimer's disease (Clarke et al., 1998). Because these conditions may need long periods of development before symptoms appear, nutritional adequacy over a lifetime becomes important. Since folate enrichment of bread and cereal products became mandatory in the United States in 1998 for the prevention of neural tube defects in newborns, an added benefit may be the protection it gives to later life diseases. Adequate intakes of vitamins B12 and B6 are important cofactors in the regulation of blood levels of homocysteine (Selhub, Bagley, Miller, & Rosenberg, 2000).

Antioxidants. These are constituents in foods, some of which have both vitamin and antioxidant activity, while others function primarily as antioxidants. Antioxidants act within the cells to prevent oxidative activity that may cause damage to other cell constituents, including DNA. A large body of evidence shows that free radicals and other oxidative molecules can cause damage that may lead to the development of some cancers, cardiovascular diseases, Parkinson's disease, and Alzheimer's disease (Ames, Shigenaga, & Hagen, 1993; Christen, 2000; Meydani, 2001; Smith, Rottkamp, Nunomura, Raina, & Perry, 2000). This damage can occur over a long period of time, and we are learning that lifelong consumption of fruits and vegetables offers the best protection from oxidative damage (Halliwell, 2000; Martin, Youdim, Szprengiel, Shukin-Hale, & Joseph, 2002). Recent reports have indicated that high dietary intake of vitamins C and E may lower the risk of Alzheimer's disease (Engelhart et al., 2002; Morris et al., 2002).

At the University Memory and Aging Center of Case Western Reserve University and University Hospitals of Cleveland, we are investigating adult lifetime risk factors for Alzheimer's disease in a case control study. Using the self-administered Life History Questionnaire, we are obtaining medical, occupational, activity, education, smoking, and food frequency histories from the surrogates of cases of persons with Alzheimer's disease as well as from healthy controls. The questionnaire focuses on three age periods: 20–39 years, 40–59 years, and 60+ years. In the Food Frequency Questionnaire, respondents indicated how often they consumed each of 98 foods during each age period. Responses were analyzed for daily consumption of nutrients and for food patterns. As shown in Table 5.1, antioxidant nutrients consumed over time may be protective for the development of Alzheimer's disease. The best food sources of antioxidants are fruits and vegetables with a variety of colors; for instance, red, yellow, green, and orange.

NUTRITION AND COGNITIVE ABILITY

Several individual nutrients and food substances have been found to be related to cognitive ability and, indeed, may be associated with reduced risk for dementias and Alzheimer's disease (Meydani, 2001; Rosenberg & Miller, 1992). We have already discussed both the effects of oxidative stress and the preventive effects of dietary antioxidants. Single dietary components that have been reported to be important in maintaining cognitive performance in aging include vitamins C, E, B12, B6, folate, and glucose and other carbohydrates (Christen, 2000; Greenwood, 2003; Tangney, 2001).

GENE-DIET INTERACTIONS

A large body of evidence shows that gene-diet interactions influence health outcomes (Simopoulos, 1999). We are just beginning to understand how genetic variation may affect food choices and dietary interventions. Aging, with the influence of chronic health conditions and medications, along with genetic variation, certainly

TABLE 5.1   Mean Consumption of Kilocalories and Selected Antioxidants*

	Cases n = 140	Controls n = 282	*P* value
Total kilocalories per day	2,127	1974	.024
Percent kilocalories from fat	38.1	37.7	NS
Nutrients per 1000 kilocalories:			
Vitamin A (RE)	849	984	<.001
Vitamin C (mg)	73.5	84.7	.002
Vitamin E (αTE)	5.5	6	NS
Pro-A carotene (mcg)	2,186	2789	<.001
Alpha Carotene (mcg)	287	384	<.001
Beta carotene (mcg)	1,876	2370	<.001
Lycopene (mcg)	696	953	<.001
Lutein (mcg)	924	1235	<.001

*Nutrients consumed over the age periods 20–39 years and 40–59 years; controlled for age, gender, and years of education Analysis of Covariance (ANCOVA).

may affect not only the taste of food, but, in turn, may affect food choices and quality of the diet (Duffy & Bartoshuk, 2000). Gene-diet interactions in obesity are being studied. While it is well understood that we cannot overcome the first law of thermodynamics, which informs us that the energy that goes in must equal the energy that comes out, we are cognizant of the fact that many Americans are becoming less active and are consuming more calories than they are expending. Thus, there is an epidemic of obesity. Genetic factors may be responsible in some persons for determining susceptibility to gaining or losing weight. These need to be identified early in life in order to determine susceptibility to the risk of developing obesity in later life. Much more research is needed to determine the genes involved and their actions (Perusse & Bouchard, 2000).

Current research is beginning to identify genotypes that may be associated with specific dietary components. Polymorphism at the apolipoprotein E (APOE) locus is responsible for variations in blood lipid responses to dietary fat interventions. It is associated with the development of atherosclerosis and with Alzheimer's disease and possibly other dementias (Berglund, 2001). The APOE epsilon 4 genotype has been determined to be a risk factor for Alzheimer's disease. However, many persons who have this genotype do not develop Alzheimer's disease. Dietary studies of persons with the different APOE genotypes (epsilon 2, 3, or 4) have focused on total calories, dietary fat, fatty acids, antioxidants, vitamins, and foods and food groups as being either risky or protective (Luchsinger, Tang, Shea, & Mayeaux, 2002; Martin et al., 2002; Masson, McNeill, & Avenell, 2003; Morris et al., 2002). In our studies, we were able to demonstrate that more of those healthy persons in the control group and with the epsilon 4 genotype consumed diets in the lowest third of fat intake. Thus, lower fat intakes may protect them from developing Alzheimer's disease in the future (Petot, 2003).

We conducted a food pattern analysis to describe food consumption patterns associated with risk for Alzheimer's disease. When food frequencies during the 40–59 year age period for cases and controls were analyzed using factor analysis, two major dietary patterns were identified. The first factor was loaded heavily with red meats, processed meats, french fries, refined grains, sweets, eggs, fried chicken, high-fat dairy products, high-energy drinks, snacks, nuts, margarine, and cold breakfast cereal. This factor was labeled as the low antioxidant-high fat diet pattern. The second factor was characterized by a high intake of fruit, vegetables, vegetable soups, whole grains, tomatoes, seafood, and poultry. This factor was labeled as the high antioxidant-low fat pattern (Table 5.2). It can be seen that the high antioxidant-low fat pattern, which includes more fruits and vegetables, represents a diet that is similar to those being recommended for all Americans as preventive for cardiovascular diseases, diabetes, and cancer. When we calculated the odds ratios for Alzheimer's disease for these diet patterns and adjusted for APOE epsilon 4, the odds ratios for Alzheimer's disease were sharply reduced (Fig. 5.1). Therefore, the advice to all is to reduce total fat, use plant oils, lower consumption of red meat, and increase fish, poultry, fruits, and vegetables. The near future may include the provision of diet counseling to accommodate genetic variation among individuals.(Blundell & Cooling, 1999; Patterson, Eaton, & Potter, 1999).

NUTRITION AND THE METABOLIC SYNDROME

The metabolic syndrome has been described as a constellation of factors associated with risk of developing cardiovascular disease. These factors include older age, hypertension, low level of HDL cholesterol, high triglyceride levels, high plasma glucose, and obe-

TABLE 5.2   Major Factors (Diet Patterns) Identified by the Factor Analysis Process*

Food or food group	Factor 1 Low antioxidant/ High fat diet pattern	Factor 2 High antioxidant/ Low fat diet pattern
Red meats	0.662	—
Sweets, desserts	0.569	—
French fries	0.568	—
Refined grains	0.557	—
Processed meats	0.509	—
Eggs	0.478	—
Fried chicken	0.448	—
High-fat dairy products	0.439	—
High-energy drinks	0.375	—
Margarine	0.369	—
Snacks	0.365	—
Nuts	0.350	—
Cold breakfast cereal	0.306	—
Chowder, cream soups	—	0.684
Poultry	—	0.681
Yellow and green vegetables	—	0.641
Fish, seafood	—	0.621
Fruit	—	0.532
Homemade, ready-made soups	—	0.518
Whole grains	—	0.488
Tomatoes	—	0.466
Other vegetables	—	0.452

*Foods or food groups with factor loadings <0.30 for both factors were excluded.

sity (Yong-Woo et al., 2003). Dietary habits throughout life will play a role in the prevention or development of these chronic conditions. Currently, there is controversy regarding the optimum dietary patterns of fat, kinds of fat, carbohydrate, and protein. Consensus on these issues is needed for the development of public policies for dietary guidance and education (Gifford, 2002).

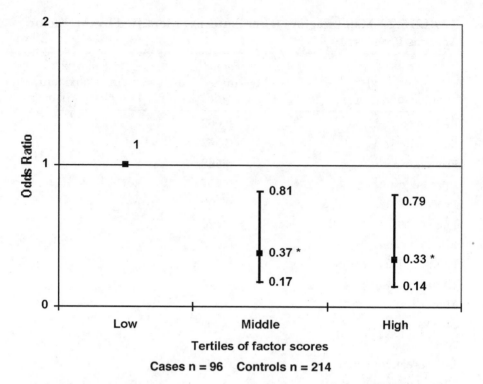

FIGURE 5.1   Odds ratios with confidence intervals for Alzheimer's disease with high antioxidant/low fat diet pattern.[a]

[a]Adjusted for year of birth, education, gender, total energy, and ApoE e4 genotype.
*$p = < .01$

NUTRITION AND QUALITY OF LIFE IN OLDER ADULTS

Health-related quality of life becomes very important as many older persons are affected by chronic health problems. Dietary habits and patterns developed over a lifetime do change over time with changing life circumstances. Age-associated body composition changes leading to reduced muscle mass and increased body fat may be attributed to reduced physical activity. A number of longitudinal studies have reported that higher intensity physical activities decline with older age (DiPietro, 2001). Reduced energy expenditure can result in increased body weight for many individuals in whom dietary reductions in calories are not made. When fewer calories are required to maintain a healthy body weight, it becomes more difficult to include all of the necessary nutrients. This introduces the concept of nutrient density—that is, the inclusion of more nutrients in fewer calories. For example, fats and oils, sugars, and starches contain many calories, but few nutrients; whereas fruits and vegetables contain few calories but are rich in nutrients. In addition, many lifestyle changes during older adulthood may have important effects on appetite and food choices. Social conditions for the enjoyment of eating are important, along with the ability to obtain and prepare food (de Castro, 2002). The presence of disease and use of medications also may alter food habits. There has been a relaxation of many dietary restrictions for the very old and frail elderly. It no longer seems prudent to impose sodium, cholesterol, or other restrictions, as they tend to reduce appetite and the intake of important nutrients (Dorner, Niedert, & Welch, 2002).

NUTRIENT SUPPLEMENTS AND HERBAL PRODUCTS

The use of nutrient supplements has become more prevalent in recent years, especially by people age 50 years or older. It is scarcely possible to ignore the advertising in the media and on the internet for a wide variety of nutrient supplements and herbal preparations (Kava, Meister, Whelan, Lukachko, & Mirabile, 2002). The Dietary Supplement Health and Education Act of 1994 defines dietary supplements as products intended to supplement the diet and containing one or more of the following; vitamin, mineral, herb, or other botanical, amino acid, dietary substance to supplement the diet by increasing the total dietary intake such as in concentrate, metabolite, constituent, extract. They are labeled as dietary supplements without claims for disease prevention, treatment, or cure (Thomson et al., 2002). It is important to note that this act does not require manufacturers to ensure safety and efficacy, nor does it require review by the USDA. This does not mean that all nutrient supplements are not to be trusted. Be sure to purchase multivitamin-mineral or calcium supplements that have a well-known brand name. There is strong evidence that many products do have health benefits; however, when purchasing single nutrient or herbal products, it is wise to consult with a health care provider, because, among other things, nutrient-nutrient and drug-nutrient interactions may interfere with the benefits (Davidson & Geohas, 2003; Fairfield & Fletcher, 2002).

NUTRITION RECOMMENDATIONS
FOR SUCCESSFUL AGING

"You are what you eat." We do not know the source of this old axiom, but we are accumulating much evidence that this is true. The environments in which we live, our genetic makeup, the lifestyles we choose, and the foods we eat can all contribute to successful aging-beginning early and continuing throughout life. Diets are only a factor, but they are a vitally important factor in determining how aging can be successful.

We are deluged with diet recommendations. *The Food Guide Pyramid* and the *U.S. Dietary Guidelines for Americans* have been published by the United States Departments of Agriculture, and Health and Human Services for over 50 years and are revised periodically (USDA & USDHHS, 2000). They are designed to provide food guidance for all healthy persons of all ages and have been found to be very good guidelines for everyone. Recent diet surveys, designed to examine the relationship of dietary patterns of different groups of people with chronic diseases and mortality, are indicating that these guideline continue to be excellent advice. Survey findings indicate that following the guidelines is associated with reduced risk for cancer, cardiovascular diseases, dementia, Alzheimer's disease, and mortality (Bazzano et al., 2002; Fung, Willett, Stampfer, Manson, & Hu, 2001; Harnack, Nicodemus, Jacobs, & Folsom, 2002; Kant, Schatzkin, Graubard, & Schairer, 2000; Michels & Wolk, 2002). Dietary patterns do change with age. Reduced energy expenditure can result in a reduction of 600–1,200 daily calorie intakes. With lower calorie requirements, there is a reduction in nutrients. Thus, it becomes more difficult to include all of the needed nutrients in a reduced-calorie pattern. For some nutrients, older persons are consuming one fifth to one third of the recommended daily intakes (Morley, 2001; Wakimoto & Block, 2001). The USDA Human Research Center on Aging at Tufts University has published a modified food guide for people over 70 years of age (Rasmussen & Lichenstein, 1999). Additions to the pyramid include an emphasis on 8 or more servings of water and the use of calcium, vitamin D, and vitamin B12 supplements after checking with a health care professional. Both of the dietary guidelines are excellent tools for recognizing that all foods can fit into a nutritious daily plan—there are no all good nor all bad foods. For everyone, moderation in all things throughout life, including diet, is the key to successful aging.

REFERENCES

Ames, B. N., Shigenaga, M. K., & Hagen, T. M. (1993). Oxidants, antioxidants, and the degenerative diseases of aging. *Proceedings of the National Academy of Science, 90*(17), 7915–7922.

Anderson, R. N. (2002). Deaths: Leading causes for 2000. *National Vital Statistics Reports, 50*(16), 1–86.

Bazzano, L. A., He, J., Ogden, L. G., Loria, C. M., Vupputuri, S., Myers, L., & Whelton, P. K. (2002). Fruit and vegetable intake and risk of cardiovascular disease in US adults: The first National Health and Nutrition Examination Survey Epidemiologic follow-up study. *American Journal of Clinical Nutrition, 76*(1), 93–99.

Berglund, L. (2001). The APOE gene and diets—food (and drink) for thought. *American Journal of Clinical Nutrition, 73,* 669–670.

Blundell, J. E., & Cooling, J. (1999). High-fat and low–fat (behavioral) phenotypes: Biology or environment? *Proceedings of the Nutrition Society, 58*(4), 773–777.

Casadesus, G., Shukitt-Hale, B., & Joseph, J. A. (2002). Qualitative versus quantitative caloric intake: Are they equivalent paths to successful aging? *Neurobiology of Aging, 23*(5), 747–769.

Christen, Y. (2000). Oxidative stress and Alzheimer disease. *American Journal of Clinical Nutrition, 71*(Suppl.), 621S–629S.

Clarke, R., Smith, A. D., Jobst, K. A., Refsum, H., Sutton, L., & Ueland, P. M. (1998). Folate, vitamin B12, and serum total homocysteine levels in confirmed Alzheimer disease. *Archives of Neurology, 55*(11), 1449–1455.

Davidson, M. H., & Geohas, C. T. (2003). Efficacy of over-the-counter nutritional supplements. *Current Atheroscler Report, 5*(1), 15–21.

Dawson-Hughes, B., & Harris, S. S. (2002). Calcium intake influences the association of protein intake with rates of bone loss in elderly men and women. *American Journal of Clinical Nutrition, 75*(4), 773–779.

de Castro, J. M. (2002). Age-related changes in social, psychological, and temporal influences on food intake in free-living, healthy, adult humans. *Journal of Gerontology: Medical Sciences, 57A*(N0 6), M368–M377.

DiPietro, L. (2001). Physical activity in aging: Changes in patterns and their relationship to health and function. *Journals of Gerontology Series A Biological Sciences and Medical Sciences, 56A*(Spec. No. 2), 13–22.

Dorner, B., Niedert, K. C., & Welch, P. K. (2002). Position of the American Dietetic Association: Liberalized diets for older adults in long–term care. *Journal of the American Dietetic Association, 102*(9), 1316–1323.

Duffy, V. B., & Bartoshuk, L. M. (2000). Food acceptance and genetic variation in taste. *Journal of the American Dietetic Association, 100*(6), 647–655.

Engelhart, M. J., Geerlings, M. I., Ruitenberg, A., van Swieten, J. C., Hofman, A., Witteman, J. C. M., & Breteler, M. M. (2002). Dietary intake of antioxidants and risk of Alzheimer disease. *Journal of the American Medical Association, 287*(24), 3223–3229.

Fairfield, K. M., & Fletcher, R. H. (2002). Vitamins for chronic disease prevention in adults. Scientific Review. *Journal of the American Medical Association, 287*(23), 3116–3126.

Fung, T. T., Willett, W. C., Stampfer, M. J., Manson, J. E., & Hu, F. B. (2001). Dietary patterns and the risk of coronary heart disease in women. *Archives of Internal Medicine, 161*(15), 1857–1862.

Gifford, K. D. (2002). Dietary fats, eating guides, and public policy: History, critique, and recommendations. *American Journal of Medicine, 113*(9B), 89S–106S.

Greenwood, C. E. (2003). Dietary carbohydrate, glucose regulation, and cognitive performance in elderly persons. *Nutrition Reviews, 61*(5 (II)), S68–S74.

Halliwell, B. (2000). Why and how should we measure oxidative DNA damage in nutritional studies? How far have we come? *American Journal of Clinical Nutrition, 72,* 1082–1087.

Harnack, L., Nicodemus, K., Jacobs, D. R., Jr., & Folsom, A. R. (2002). An evaluation of the dietary guidelines for Americans in relation to cancer occurrence. *American Journal of Clinical Nutrition, 76*(4), 889–896.

Jacobsen, D. W. (1998). Homocysteine and vitamins in cardiovascular disease. *Clinical Chemistry, 44,* 1833–1834.

Kant, K. K., Schatzkin, A., Graubard, B. I., & Schairer, C. (2000). A prospective study of diet quality and mortality in women. *Journal of the American Medical Association, 283,* 2109–2115.

Kava, R., Meister, K. A., Whelan, E. M., Lukachko, A. M., & Mirabile, C. (2002). Dietary supplement: Safety information in magazines popular among older readers. *Journal of Health Communication, 7*(1), 13–23.

Koplan, J. P., & Fleming, D. W. (2000). Current and future public health challenges. *Journal of the American Medical Association, 284*(13), 1696–1698.

Luchsinger, J. A., Tang, M.-X., Shea, S., & Mayeaux, R. (2002). Caloric intake and the risk of Alzheimer disease. *Archives of Neurology, 59*(8), 1258–1263.

Martin, A., Youdim, K., Szprengiel, A., Shukin-Hale, B., & Joseph, J. (2002). Roles of Vitamins E and C on neurodegenerative diseases and cognitive performance. *Nutrition Reviews, 60*(11), 308–334.

Masoro, E. J. (2000). Caloric restriction and aging. *Experimental Gerontology, 35,* 299–305.

Masson, L. F., McNeill, G., & Avenell, A. (2003). Genetic variation and the lipid response to dietary intervention: A systematic review. *American Journal of Clinical Nutrition, 77*(5), 1098–1111.

Meydani, M. (2001). Antioxidants and cognitive function. *Nutrition Review, 59*(8), (II)S75–S82.

Michels, K. B., & Wolk, A. (2002). A prospective study of variety of healthy foods and mortality in women. *International Journal of Epidemiology, 31*(4), 847–854.

Morley, J. E. (2001). Decreased food intake with aging. *Journal of Gerontology, Series A, 56A*(Special Issue II), 81–88.

Morris, M. C., Evans, D. A., Bienias, J. L., Tangney, C. C., Bennett, D. A., Aggarwal, N., Wilson, R. S., & Scherr, P. A. (2002). Dietary intake of antioxidant nutrients and the risk of incident Alzheimer disease in a biracial community study. *Journal of the American Medical Association, 287*(24), 3230–3237.

Nicolas, A.-S., Andrieu, S., Nourhashemi, F., Rolland, Y., & Vellas, B. (2001). Successful aging and nutrition. *Nutrition Review, 59*(8), (II)S88–S92.

Nielson, S. J., & Popkin, B. M. (2003). Patterns and trends in food portion sizes, 1977–1998. *Journal of the American Medical Association, 289*(4), 450–453.

Patterson, R. E., Eaton, D. L., & Potter, J. D. (1999). The genetic revolution: Change and challenge for the dietetics profession. *Journal of the American Dietetic Association, 99*(11), 1412–1420.

Perusse, L., & Bouchard, C. (2000). Gene-diet interactions in obesity. *American Journal of Clinical Nutrition, 72*(Suppl.), 1285S–1290S.

Petot, G. J. (2003). Interactions of apolipoprotein E genotype and dietary fat intake of healthy older persons during mid-adult life. *Metabolism, 52*(3), 279–281.

Rosenberg, I. H., & Miller, J. W. (1992). Nutritional factors in physical and cognitive functions of elderly people. *American Journal of Clinical Nutrition, 55*(6 suppl.), 1237S–1243S.

Roth, G. S. (2001). Caloric restriction in primates and relevance to humans. *Annals of the New York Academy of Sciences, 928*, 305–315.

Russell, R.M., Rasmussen, H., & Lichtenstein, A. H. (1999). Modified food guide pyramid for people over seventy years of age. *Journal of Nutrition, 129*(3), 751–753.

Selhub, J., Bagley, L. C., Miller, J., & Rosenberg, I. H. (2000). B vitamins, homocysteine, and neurocognitive function in the elderly. *American Journal of Clinical Nutrition, 71*(2), 614S–620S.

Simopoulos, A. P. (1999). Genetic variation and nutrition. *Nutrition Review, 57*(5), (II)S10–S19.

Smith, M. A., Rottkamp, C. A., Nunomura, A., Raina, A. K., & Perry, G. (2000). Oxidative stress in Alzheimer's disease. *Biochimica et Biophysics Acta, 1502*(1), 139–144.

Tangney, C. C. (2001). Does vitamin E protect against cognitive changes as we age? *Nutrition, 17*(10), 806–808.

Thomson, C., Diekman, C., Fragakis, A. S., Meershaert, C., Holler, H., & Devlin, C. (2002). Guidelines regarding the recommendation and sale of dietary supplements. *Journal of the American Dietetic Association, 102*(8), 1158–1164.

USDA, & USDHHS. (2000). *Dietary guidelines for Americans, 5th ed.* Washington, DC: US Department of Agriculture, US Department of Health and Human Services.

Wakimoto, P., & Block, G. (2001). Dietary intake, dietary patterns, and changes with age: An epidemiological perspective. *Journal of Gerontology, Series A, 56A*(Special Issue II), 65–80.

Weindruch, R., & Sohal, R. S. (1997). Caloric intake and aging. *New England Journal of Medicine, 337*(14), 986–994.

Yong-Woo, P., Zhu, S., Palaniappan, L., Heshka, S., Carnethon, M., & Heymsfield, S. B. (2003). The metabolic syndrome. *Archives of Internal Medicine, 163,* 427–436.

Young, L. R., & Nestle, M. (2003). Expanding portion sizes in the US marketplace: Implications for nutrition counseling. *Journal of the American Dietetic Association, 103*(2), 231–234.

CHAPTER 6

Successful Aging in the Face of Chronic Disease

Eva Kahana, Cathie King, Boaz Kahana, Heather Menne, Noah J. Webster, Amy Dan, Kyle Kercher, Alexandra Bohne, and Carolyn Lechner

Successful aging represents a positive development in gerontological theorizing, for it has shifted the focus away from viewing older adults as a dependent group whose problems tax the resources of society to considering the contributing potential of older adults. This shift has been labeled as a move from dependency to autonomy or agency-based models of aging (Midlarsky & Kahana, 1994). The emphasis on successful aging or aging well helps dispel negative stereotypes and removes some of the stigma associated with being an aged person. Models of successful aging have sought to understand the resources and behaviors that facilitate aging well and typically point to the maintenance of healthy lifestyles as deterrents to chronic illness and attendant impairments (Rowe & Kahn, 1998). Behind the optimistic message of these models of successful aging, however, there lies an exclusionary orientation, whereby chronically ill and disabled older adults do not have a place at the table of successful aging. This chapter articulates a model of successful aging we developed (Kahana & Kahana, 1996; 2003; Kahana, Kahana, & Kercher, in press), which allows for understanding criteria of successful aging that are based on human agency and are particularly salient for the many older persons facing the challenges of chronic illness.

It is particularly important to study how older people can cope with chronic disease, because over 100 million Americans have chronic health problems (Robert Wood Johnson Foundation, 1996), with rates of chronic disease increasing with age. The prevalence of chronic health problems will continue to grow as people live longer and as the large cohort of baby boomers ages in upcoming years. Chronic health problems have negative consequences for both individuals and for society. Chronic disease can lead to disability, additional health problems, and reduced quality of life (Jette, 1996; National Center for Chronic Disease Prevention and Health Promotion, 2002). Of those who have a chronic health problem, one third of those ages 65–74 and 45% of those ages 75 and older are limited in their activities because of health problems (National Academy on an Aging Society, 1999). Furthermore, in 1995, it was estimated that medical care costs for Americans with chronic conditions was $470 billion (Robert Wood Johnson Foundation, 1996).

MODEL OF SUCCESSFUL AGING

Our model of successful aging, termed preventive and corrective proactivity, has been described in detail in our previous publications (Kahana & Kahana, 1996; 2003; Kahana, Kahana, & Kercher, in press). Here we provide only a very brief synopsis of principles of the model and then turn to a discussion about the ways in which criteria of success advocated in the model can apply to older adults facing a variety of common chronic illnesses.

As sociologists, we must be particularly cognizant that social contextual factors, such as ethnic/racial background and access to medical care, have an impact on older persons' life opportunities and choices (Link & Phelan, 1995), including their propensity to develop chronic disease. In the psychological literature, successful adaptation in the face of stressful life events or chronic stressors has been conceptualized in the framework of resilience (Carstensen & Freud, 1994). Discussions related to maintenance of the aging self are focused on cognitive maneuvers, such as changes in goal salience. While our model of successful aging recognizes that psychological dispositions (such as hopefulness and self-esteem) may impact both on proactive adaptations and quality of life outcomes, we conceptualize proactive adaptations in behavioral rather than cognitive terms.

Our comprehensive model of Successful Aging (Fig. 6.1) specifies how the stressors (component B) of chronic illness, long-term and recent life events, and person-environment incongruence, in the absence of ameliorative buffers, set off a chain of events leading to adverse quality of life outcomes (component F). This model reflects traditional hypotheses about the role of internal resources (component C) and external resources (component E) in ameliorating adverse stress effects. Our model also emphasizes the buffering roles of proactive behaviors (component D) in reducing (moderating) the adverse consequences of stressors on quality of life, and recognizes the influences of both the temporal and spatial context (component A). We propose that spatial influences (demographic characteristics and community) and temporal context (history and biography) will have main effects on each of the stressors, buffers, and quality of life outcome components of our model. Presentation of our conceptual model has been simplified by focusing on unidirectional causal linkages. We recognize, however, that alternative directions of causality are often plausible and may be tested in longitudinal studies utilizing the proposed model.

In our model of successful aging, we acknowledge the important roles played by both external and internal resources (components C and E in our model). Such psychological, financial, social, and environmental resources are well-accepted buffers in the context of the stress paradigm (Pearlin, Lieberman, Menaghan, & Mullan, 1981). In the present discussion, our major focus is on the unique cornerstone of our model, describing behavioral adaptations termed preventive and corrective proactivity. In our orientation to buffers in our proactivity model (Fig. 6.1), we view older adults as active agents who engage in preventive and corrective behaviors to maximize their quality of life in the face of stressors, such as chronic illness. These proactive efforts are facilitated by possessing both external and internal resources.

In this chapter, we focus on the most salient components of our model for understanding successful aging in the face of chronic illness. We hone in on some chronic illnesses that constitute normative stressors of aging and focus primarily on proactive behavioral adaptations as factors that can buffer the adverse effects of chronic illness on quality of life. Nevertheless, most older people suffer

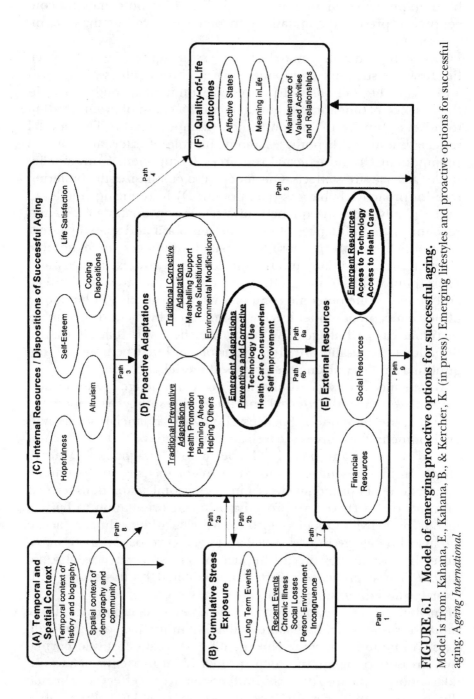

FIGURE 6.1   Model of emerging proactive options for successful aging.

Model is from: Kahana, E., Kahana, B., & Kercher, K. (in press). Emerging lifestyles and proactive options for successful aging. *Ageing International.*

from multiple chronic conditions and, hence, our discussion based on single conditions reflects a simplified analysis of the issues they confront daily.

Preventive Adaptations

While our discussion of specific chronic diseases focuses on corrective adaptations useful after the onset of illnesses, preventive adaptations do play an important role in forestalling the occurrence of several major chronic diseases.

Health Promotion. A sedentary lifestyle and obesity have been shown to be major risk factors in the onset of health problems, including diabetes and cardiovascular disease (Miller, Balady, & Fletcher, 1997; Shirey & Summer, 2000). Alternatively engaging in exercise and good dietary habits are major preventive efforts that can help delay the onset of these life-threatening conditions. Individuals who have strong family histories of specific chronic conditions might place special emphasis on health promoting lifestyles, as well as on seeking health screening for early detection of those health conditions.

Planning Ahead. Planning ahead is a preventive adaptation helpful for coping with chronic disease. Planning ahead for potential care needs prior to the onset of an illness can be highly beneficial. Thus, for example, it is both more feasible and affordable to purchase long-term care insurance prior to the diagnosis of a chronic illness so that older adults retain the possibility of continuing to live in their own homes and receive necessary care after being diagnosed with serious chronic illnesses. Financial planning can help ensure that one has adequate resources for retirement living and can purchase assistive devices or services, such as hiring a driver. While proactive strategies of planning ahead may not be able to prevent the emergence of chronic disease, they can help build financial and social resources, which can assist after illness has set in.

Helping Others. Helping others prior to the onset of chronic disease can also serve to build an older individual's social resources from which he or she can benefit after the onset of chronic illness. Indeed our own research (Kahana & Borawski, 1997) has documented that those older adults who have provided aid to friends while they were in good health subsequently obtained more assistance from friends in general after they had become ill. It should be noted that such help was not necessarily received from the individuals to whom elders had initially provided aid.

Corrective Adaptations

We provide a detailed discussion of the potential usefulness of specific corrective adaptations proposed in our successful aging model as we discuss illustrative examples of specific chronic illnesses. Here we offer a general overview of the corrective adaptations posited in our model.

Marshalling Support. Marshalling support refers to efforts by older adults to request assistance from informal or formal sources. Marshalling support is successfully contingent both on the willingness to disclose problems (Pennebacker, 1995) and the availability of sources of social support (Antonucci & Akiyama, 1991). Older adults generally turn to family and friends for support prior to seeking and accepting help from formal sources (Cantor, 1979). In terms of marshalling support relevant to chronic illnesses, such requests may range from seeking help with transportation to physician appointments to actual caregiving tasks specifically related to an illness, such as administration of medications or watching for the safety of a cognitively impaired older person. Formal help seeking can range from utilizing physician's services to seeking aid from other professionals, such as psychologists or physical therapists, and finally extends to hiring of paid helpers or utilizing assistance offered by diverse service agencies.

Role Substitution. Role substitution in our model of successful aging was originally used to demonstrate alternative social roles undertaken by individuals as they experience social losses due to life events, such as widowhood or involuntary retirement. However, in the context of chronic illness, role substitution assumes special salience. Older adults may have difficulty performing usual roles, such as worker or homemaker, because of the physical impairments experienced due to chronic illness. Even when a social role, such as that of spouse, grandparent, or friend, is not formally affected, the chronically ill person must take proactive steps to modify or substitute activities as they enact a given role. The wife with heart disease who finds cooking too stressful due to chronic illness may substitute other contributions, such as paying bills or other more sedentary tasks, to continue enacting her role. Similarly, the grandparent who can no longer drive grandchildren to baseball games may substitute playing checkers or bingo.

Activity and Environmental Modifications. Activity and environmental modifications are highly salient proactive adaptations for the chronically ill elderly. They reflect adaptations that are designed to reduce the demand on an impaired older person and may involve use of assistive devices to help accomplish desired activities (Lawton, 1990). Activity or environmental modifications can also be used to enhance the comfort or safety of an older person. Older adults often initiate corrective environmental and activity modifications that help increase their autonomy or comfort and go beyond safety-conscious environmental changes generally recommended by professionals (Kahana, King, Brown, DeCrane, Mackey, Monaghan, Raff, Wu, Kercher, & Stange, 1994). It is noteworthy that older adults have found those assistive devices that are widely used by the general population (such as big button phones) less stigmatizing than special devices aimed at the aged. Our own research has confirmed that assistive device use significantly diminishes the adverse effects of chronic illness and physical impairment on the quality of life of the elderly (Kahana, Chirayath, Wisniewski, Kahana, & Kercher, 2003).

Emergent Adaptations

In the development of our successful aging model, we have recently introduced consideration of emergent proactive adaptations, which present new options for coping with stressors faced by the chronically ill elderly of the 21st century (Kahana, Kahana, & Kercher, in press). As shown in our model (component D), these include technology use, health care consumerism, and self-improvement.

Technology Use. Advanced technologies, including cellular phones, the internet, and health monitoring devices, offer new sources of empowerment by enhancing information, communication, and self-care abilities of chronically ill older adults (Thursz, Nusberg, & Prather, 1995). Older adults whose mobility is limited may benefit greatly by making social contacts and even marshalling support via e-mail (Lawhon & Ennis, 1995). The ability to obtain medical information and discuss medical conditions and seek advice from others having similar problems through the internet may be particularly useful for older adults afflicted with multiple and changing chronic conditions (White et al., 1999). Telemedicine is increasingly prevalent as a health care resource, allowing health monitoring and communication with health care providers (Starren et al., 2002).

Health Care Consumerism. It has been increasingly recognized that in the era of managed care, patients can benefit from playing an active role as health care consumers by communicating proactively with health care providers and acting as advocates for themselves and those they care for (Rodwin, 1997). Health care consumerism implies both taking the initiative and being assertive in encounters with health care providers (Kahana & Kahana, 2001). Rather than assuming an adversarial approach, proactive health care consumers can work toward forging an alliance that includes the chronically ill older person, the caregiver, physician, and/or other key members of the health care team (Kahana & Kahana, 2003).

Self-Improvement. While efforts at self-improvement or self-actualization are generally associated with the well elderly, there is increasing recognition that such efforts can meaningfully benefit the chronically ill aged. Our definition of self-improvement as an emerging set of adaptations has included education, improving one's physical appearance, and seeking personal and spiritual growth. At a time when physical impairment limits many daily physical activities, having a new skill (such as playing bridge or card games with others) can serve as a most useful adaptation. Where ravages of illness or medical treatments have threatened the physical appearance of the chronically ill, special attention to clothing or other forms of grooming can help build self-esteem. As chronic illness may raise issues about longevity and mortality, seeking spiritual fulfillment may also prove to be a most useful coping strategy.

APPLICATION OF MODEL TO SPECIFIC CHRONIC CONDITIONS

Diverse chronic diseases pose some similar challenges, as well as some unique ones. Similarly, the corrective adaptations that may help older individuals to deal with these stressors successfully also have overlapping, as well as unique, aspects. There are differences in the challenges faced by patients dealing with the same illness depending on the length of time they had it, on illness severity, and on treatment requirements. It should also be noted that expectations for positive outcomes among different dimensions of quality of life are likely to differ based on illness characteristics.

Even as we recognize these complexities, for illustrative purposes, we present in this chapter examples of four prevalent chronic diseases with which older adults typically cope. Specifically, we focus on arthritis (the most prevalent chronic illness faced by older adults), cardiovascular disease, diabetes, and early-stage dementia. We should note that we have addressed unique challenges and successes in coping with cancer (Kahana, Kahana, & Deimling, 2002) and HIV/AIDs in separate articles (e.g., Kahana & Kahana, 2001).

Subsequent to presenting illustrations of the four chronic diseases on which we focus, we will provide some case studies of older adults who have participated in our longitudinal study of adaptation to frailty in late life, which gave rise to our conceptualization of successful aging. (For a detailed description of our study sample and selected study findings, see Borawksi, Kinney, & Kahana, 1996; and Kahana et al., 2002). These case studies elucidate the many creative ways older adults can maintain psychological well-being, a positive sense of self, and meaning in life even as they face multiple chronic illnesses.

Arthritis

Arthritis is the most common chronic health problem among adults aged 65 and older (Desai, Ahang, & Hennessy, 1999; National Academy on an Aging Society, 1999), with osteoarthritis being the most prevalent type of arthritis. Symptoms of arthritis can include joint inflammation, fatigue, pain, and stiffness. Arthritis can lead to decreased mobility and functioning (Boult, Kane, Louis, Boult, & McCaffrey, 1994; Downe-Wamboldt & Melanson, 1998), loss of independence, and feelings of helplessness (Burckhardt, 1988). While medications are available to help relieve arthritis pain, reduce inflammation, and improve functioning (Panush & Holtz, 1994; The Arthritis Foundation, 2002), there is no cure for arthritis. However, individuals can use several different strategies to manage their arthritis symptoms.

Regular exercise (classified as health promotion or primarily a preventive strategy in our model) can help strengthen muscles and bones and improve symptoms of arthritis, such as reducing pain and improving functioning. Some physicians recommend that arthritis patients visit with occupational or physical therapists to assist them in their therapy or to help establish exercise regimens. In addition, many patients with arthritis visit complementary and alternative practitioners, such as podiatrists, who may also recommend various exercises and strategies to alleviate negative symptoms (Kaboli, Doebbeling, Saag, & Rosenthal, 2001). Range-of-motion and endurance exercises are often suggested for arthritis. Swimming is a popular activity arthritis patients engage in to relieve symptoms, while remaining physically active. Alternative exercises, like yoga, massages, and relaxation techniques (e.g., prayer and use of relaxation tapes) can be used to help relieve and relax painful areas. Cognitive coping maneuvers (reflecting dispositional strategies in the model), including thinking positive and not focusing on the pain, are also recommended (The Arthritis Foundation, 2002).

Individuals with arthritis can benefit from corrective strategies whereby they modify their activities to reduce negative symptoms. Examples of modifications include avoiding remaining in one position for a long period of time, learning the proper way to move to reduce pain and avoid injury, not overdoing it when beginning to experience pain, and avoiding activities that hurt affected areas (The Arthritis Foundation, 2002, Horstman, 1999). To help reduce stiffness and pain, many arthritis patients use heat (e.g., heating pads or warm baths) and cold (e.g., ice packs). Individuals with arthritis also use many innovative devices to assist them, such as jar openers, reachers, grab bars, and specially designed scissors, which have been found to significantly improve their functioning and ability to complete everyday tasks (Mann, Hurren, & Tomita, 1995; Nordenskiold, 1997).

In summary, the health promoting behavior of exercise and activity and environmental modifications have been found particularly beneficial to older adults with arthritis. Assistive devices for arthritis patients, such as easy-to-open medicine bottles, are increasingly available in drug and grocery stores, making them easy for older adults to access. To the extent that such proactive adaptations are utilized, they are proven helpful in enhancing both psychological well-being and maintenance of meaningful activities and relationships as depicted in our model.

Heart Disease

Over 60 million Americans have some form of heart disease (Winters, 1997). Heart disease is one of the most common chronic conditions among individuals aged 75 and older (National Academy on an Aging Society, 1999) and is the leading cause of death in the United States (Winters, 1997). Heart disease ranges in type and has an impact on people of all ages. Older individuals are more likely to have coronary heart disease, also known· as heart attack or chest pain, which is more debilitating than other types of heart disease (National Academy on an Aging Society, 2000). The risk factors for heart disease include high blood pressure, high blood cholesterol, smoking, obesity, physical inactivity, diabetes, and stress (American Health Assistance Foundation, 2002).

A major impairment linked to heart disease is the decreased ability to perform daily tasks and activities. One study found that two out of five people aged 70 or older with heart disease required assistance with activities of daily living (Lee, O'Neill, & Summer, 2000), such as bathing, dressing, eating, using the toilet, walking, and getting into and out of bed (National Academy on an Aging Society, 2000). Heart disease among older adults has been linked to making changes in driving habits (Gallo, Rebok, & Lesikar, 1999), and in some cases causes people to retire early. Such changes can lead to a sense of helplessness and loss of independence. Those with heart disease are also more likely to become depressed (National Academy on an Aging Society, 2000).

Health promoting behaviors and having a healthy lifestyle can reduce a person's risk of getting heart disease by 80% (National Academy on an Aging Society, 2000). Individuals who are not overweight, do not smoke, consume one alcoholic drink per day, exercise on a daily basis for 30 or more minutes, and eat low-fat high-fiber diets have a considerably reduced risk of getting heart disease (National Academy on an Aging Society, 2000).

It is also recommended that those with heart disease engage in health promoting behaviors and live a healthy lifestyle. Other adaptations that can be made include marshalling the support of others, such as family members and friends, to help assist in performing daily tasks that may become difficult as a result of heart disease. Modifications can also be made to the home environment to facilitate the performance of daily tasks, such as moving necessities closer together for easier access. One example is moving the washer and dryer to the main level of the house, or moving to an apartment on the first floor where no stairs have to be used. An individual may also substitute alternative roles in their life. For example, if they are no longer able to work, they may focus more on other valued roles in their life, such as being a spouse, parent, grandparent, friend, or church member. To maintain meaningful activities and relationships in life a person may modify activities to accommodate to their heart disease. An example may be a person who enjoys taking walks with friends. This person may adjust his or her walking route to one that has more available benches so she or he can stop and rest rather than give up this activity.

Individuals who consider themselves to be at risk for heart disease can use emergent adaptations of technology, by relying on electronic heart monitors and blood-pressure counters to monitor their heart's condition and functioning. Other forms of technology can be used as corrective adaptations, such as using the Internet to order and have groceries delivered to the home. Also, efforts at self-improvement such as engaging in speech therapy or reciting poetry have been found to have a positive effect on the heart rate (Bettermann, von Bonin, Fruhwirth, Cysarz, & Moser, 2002) and can be used as a method to manage heart disease.

Diabetes

Diabetes affects 20% of the population by the age of 75 (National Academy on an Aging Society, 1999). For elderly individuals living with diabetes, proactive adaptations to promote successful aging are critical to both quality and duration of life (Meneilly & Tessier, 2001). Diabetes brings with it the threat of debilitating and potentially life-threatening side effects. Elderly diabetics are at risk for heart disease, neuropathies, retinopathy, and high blood pressure. Ultimately, diabetes can lead to amputations, heart attacks, strokes, and subsequent cognitive impairments (Rogers, 2001).

The diagnosis of diabetes, while life-saving, can add significant stressors due to treatment demands. Diabetics are required to test their blood-glucose levels. Depending on the severity of their condition, diabetes may be controlled by pills or insulin requiring injection several times a day. For an elderly individual who is possibly already taking several other medications daily, this can add a significant amount of stress.

One of the most significant corrective adaptations that a diabetic can make is to lose weight. Even a loss of 5–10% of body weight can significantly decrease the likelihood of, or reduce the severity of resultant physical health problems by increasing the efficacy of insulin absorption (Pasanisi, Contaldo, de Simone, & Mancini, 2001). The adoption of a strength-training routine can also positively impact insulin resistance by increasing muscle mass and consequently deceasing fat (Mazzeo & Tanaka, 2001). Familial support increases the likelihood that an individual will maintain his or her treatment regime, making marshalling support critical (Hurley & Roth, 2000).

Important, too, are changes in quality of life that result from a diagnosis of diabetes. Although it is not unreasonable to expect fairly good physical health outcomes if proper proactive adaptations are taken, these do not address the issue of the impact such adaptations have on everyday life. Diabetics must adapt their lifestyle by frequently measuring their blood glucose levels, injecting insulin, and sticking to a fairly strict diet and scheduled mealtimes. This loss of flexibility in the timing and content of meals has been found to negatively impact satisfaction with life, even when controlling for physical health outcomes (Bradley & Speight, 2002).

Over the past decade, a number of advances have been made that make diabetes control much simpler for individuals. Home blood-testing kits have become more sophisticated, with current digital models becoming more accurate and more portable and no longer requiring individuals to do more than write down their blood glucose levels and act accordingly. An innovative project through Columbia University has studied the use of a home telemedicine unit for diabetics that allows them to electronically transmit their blood glucose and blood-pressure readings to their physician and allows for video conferencing and Web messaging between doctor and patient. This system was found to be both cost effective and usable even by elders with no computer experience (Starren et al., 2002). Advances in artificial insulin also allow for more sophisticated control over blood glucose, allowing medications to come ever closer to approximating a normal metabolism (Liebl, 2002). Although the use of home modifications is high among diabetics, minority elders are much less likely to have these modifications, primarily due to lower financial resources (Tabbarah, Silverstein, & Seeman, 2000).

Cognitive Impairment

Cognitive impairment and cognitive decline are associated with aging and are evidenced by prevalence rates of dementia. The prevalence of dementia in the 65–70 year-old age group is 1%. This prevalence jumps to 11% for people 80–85 years old, 21% for those aged 85–90, and 39% for those aged 90–95 (Skoog, Blennow, & Marcusson, 1996). Cognitive impairment can be a significant stressor in the life of an older adult because of resulting social problems wherein the older adult has difficulty relating to others and remembering events, places, and people. These difficulties create daily limitations and may cause fear of personal or family embarrassment.

While a person with cognitive decline cannot prevent the initial decline, there are adaptations one can make to avoid or reduce problems in the future. Thinking about and planning for the future is crucial when one is experiencing cognitive decline. For instance, decisions can be made early regarding long-term care options and insurance, end-of-life choices, and, if applicable, participation in medication trials. By planning ahead, a person with cognitive decline can be assured that his or her wishes are acknowledged, and he or she can regain a sense of control in what is an often confusing time (Post & Whitehouse, 1995).

A person with cognitive decline can implement corrective adaptations as a means of maintaining his or her present state while living with the limitations imposed by the cognitive decline. A person with cognitive impairment can still marshal support to ensure that his or her best interests are enacted by either informal supports (family and friends) or by formal supports (service agencies or long-term care facilities). For example, a cognitively impaired person living in a nursing home can still be proactive by gaining the favor of the staff to make the stay at the nursing home more livable, or a cognitively impaired person can ask a cognitively intact family member to advocate for him or her when a facility is forcing the impaired person to participate in unsatisfying activities.

Role substitution is another proactive adaptation that a person with mild cognitive impairment can implement. For example, a 64-year-old retired professor diagnosed with probable Alzheimer's disease described how his social role of a classroom professor changed with his diagnosis. He detailed how he always helped people in the past and that is why he was a teacher, and now that he has had a diagnosis of Alzheimer's disease, his role has changed, but he still sees himself as a teacher. He is now helping to educate other people with cognitive impairment as to how to still maintain their life and lifestyle despite the diagnosis. In addition, he is educating researchers by participating in biological, psychological, and sociological research that explores the causes, limitations, and experiences of Alzheimer's disease (Menne, Kinney, & Morhardt, 2002).

Activity modifications for a person with cognitive impairment may include decreasing the length of trips or planning trips in greater detail than in the past. Reminder notes have been found to be useful in assisting older persons with cognitive deficits (Guerette, Nakai, Verran, & Sommerville, 1992). Personal hygiene behaviors, such as bathing and dressing, may be modified systematically so that the task can be completed in a stress-free manner. For example, a person with cognitive decline may now place his or her clothes out the night before (with or without the help of a spouse) to avoid the problem of rushing to put together a matching outfit in the morning. Another corrective adaptation that can make life easier and help one maintain a sense of independence involves meal preparation. A person with cognitive decline can still prepare simple meals on his or her own, or he or she may assist a family member by being in charge of one part of the meal, such as the salad. These modifications can continue to take place even when the person with cognitive decline is residing in a long-term care facility. A wheelchair-bound resident may be placed by well-meaning staff in a very lively activity program. If this program is too stimulating, the resident may attempt to get relief by quietly wheeling his or her chair around, leaving the group, and moving to a quiet corner of the room.

More and more, community resources are striving to meet the needs not only of the loved one of the person with cognitive decline, but with the individual as well. Agencies that once offered support to family members alone are recognizing that people living with a diagnosis are in need of caring as well and are offering groups for their participation. Sharing one's experiences with cognitive changes with others who are also coping may offer unique insights and strategies to the person, thus diminishing feelings of isolation and fear.

ILLUSTRATIVE EXAMPLES OF SUCCESSFUL AGING

We now turn to a discussion of how three older adults in our study engaged in proactive adaptations and maintained quality of life in the face of serious and worsening chronic illness.

Case 1

John began the study at age 90 (in 1989). He was a high-school graduate and had owned his own food service company. He was a widow and has three children, two of whom live in Florida. At the beginning of the study, John had arthritis and had had a hip replacement, which slightly limited the amount of walking he could do. John enjoyed many activities, including bowling, golfing, and traveling. He was proud of his health, believing he could do what most "younger men can do," and that "nothing can stop me." One of his goals was to outlive his children.

Over the 10 years he was interviewed annually, John's health declined in many ways. Three years after beginning the study, he was diagnosed with diabetes. His hip problems worsened over time to the point that he became significantly impaired in his ability to complete instrumental and personal activities of daily living. He also developed vision and sensory impairments. At age 99, he began to have memory problems, which became quite severe the year he died, in 1999.

John's positive attitude persisted throughout the course of his health decline, and he utilized multiple strategies to maintain high quality of life. He implemented many activity and environmental modifications and used assistive devices to enable maximum functioning and said he did activities in moderation to maintain his health. He had a hearing aid and used a phone amplifier for his hearing problems. For his vision problems, he wore glasses, used a magnifier, and had a big screen television. John eventually had to cut back on the amount of reading he did and had to stop driving because of vision impairments. John's hip problems resulted in greater mobility problems over the years (including difficulty walking up and down stairs and difficulty completing household tasks). John installed a handheld shower, grab bars in the bathroom, and a raised toilet seat. To enable him to get around, he used a walker and cane as needed, and had an electrical lift chair. His girlfriend and son (who lived nearby) largely provided him instrumental (e.g., transportation) and emotional support. Six years after the study began, John moved to a life-care facility in a nearby area due to a greater need for services.

In the last 2 years of his life, despite his ailing health and growing cognitive problems, John still reported high life satisfaction and low levels of depressive symptomatology. However, he began denying he had serious health problems. His son came in the mornings to prepare his breakfast and give him his medications during the last two years of his life. The annual interviewer remarked that he would have had to move to a floor that provided more assistance if he had not had his son to help him.

Case 2

Marge was 82 years old when we first interviewed her. She moved to Florida from the Midwest at age 55, after the death of her husband. She remained single throughout the balance of our study. Marge had two adult sons, one who died tragically in his mid-30s, leaving one surviving adult child. She had completed 2 years of college and never worked outside the home. Her yearly income and assets were quite small, totaling less than $10,000.

Throughout the study, Marge's chronic illnesses became more severe. At the beginning of the study, she reported having arthritis, cataracts, high blood pressure, a hiatal hernia, and tumors in her bladder. Despite all these conditions, she showed no evidence of problems with her instrumental activities of daily living. Over the next 10 years, her health declined significantly. Problems included: bladder cancer, skin cancer, mobility problems, having a hip replacement, balance troubles, incontinence, and having blood clots in her legs. Her poor health resulted in several falls over time and in significant problems with instrumental activities of daily living, but her cognitive health remained intact.

Marge was initially involved in multiple volunteer activities (including volunteering at a nursing home), had hobbies (dancing and knitting), and did exercises regularly (such as swimming). She reported no depressive symptoms but did express a desire for more companionship. Over the course of the study, coupled with growing health problems and increasingly loneliness, Marge's financial picture continued to decline. She eventually had to stop exercising due to physical limitations and had to reduce the number of hours she volunteered. As a substitute activity, she increased the amount of knitting she did, giving both knitted items to family members and multiple charities. Marge's son became divorced the second year she was in the study, and they eventually moved into a new condominium at the retirement community together. The living arrangement increased the quality of Marge's life because of the significant amount of support and companionship he provided to her, as well as sharing financial resources. Like John, Marge incorporated many devices to help her with her daily activities, including using a cane when necessary, a shower seat and hand-held shower in the bathroom, a phone amplifier, and a Lifeline device. When we last met with Marge, she was still having difficulty getting around, but she continues to devote much of her time to knitting presents.

Case 3

Tom is 90 years of age, and he entered our study at age 77. Tom was married and had two adult daughters who lived outside of Florida. Tom had been self-employed as an insurance broker. He planned well for his retirement, with his family income exceeding $50,000 a year and assets in excess of $300,000 at the time of retirement.

Tom experienced chronic eye problems throughout his life, and before entering the study, he had a heart attack. His heart problems and high blood pressure worsened over the course of the study, although he had few limitations in activities of daily living. Tom had to have bypass surgery and was diagnosed with prostate cancer. Reporting stabilizing health in the 5th year of the study, Tom took a trip and reported improved life goals and aims. After this year, his health continued to decline, until he eventually suffered from a ministroke, and then his vision problems considerably worsened. Not wanting to move to a sheltered environment, Tom and his wife marshalled support from their daughter. She eventually moved from the Midwest to Florida to help her parents.

Despite the chronic health problems, Tom always considered himself healthy compared to others his age. He lived a health-promoting lifestyle, quitting his smoking habit in his 40s, drinking only occasionally, limiting his sugar, salt, and caffeine intake, and always wearing his seatbelt. Throughout the study, Tom exercised at least three times a week and participated in numerous social activities, including golf and dining out with friends. At age 90 today, he continues to drive. Examples of continued role engagement and role substitution include his increasing volunteer activities and organization participation. As his chronic illnesses have worsened, he continues to volunteer for neighbors, participates in the rotary club, and engages in organized church activities. He considers himself religious (he attends church regularly).

These three examples demonstrate how individuals facing serious chronic conditions can take initiatives and make adaptations to their lifestyles and maintain quality of life. The cases we presented were selected not because they were exceptional individuals who were participating in our study. Rather, they were selected because they used diverse proactive adaptations from our model and had different backgrounds (different marital history, gender, financial situation, type of chronic diseases, etc.).

DISCUSSION

This chapter has described many ways older adults with chronic health problems can act to improve and maintain their quality of life. Although we focused on the agent-oriented component in our model of successful aging (proactive adaptations [component D]), our model does not exclude the importance of social structure (component A). Rather, we recognize that individuals can only make decisions about their health and life situations within the confines of their social structural positions (Hagestad & Dannefer, 2001; Settersten, 2003). We will first provide an example of how an external resource from our model affects one's abilities to engage in proactive adaptations and then move to a discussion of how larger structural forces, including laws and public policies, impact on proactivity.

As previously mentioned, internal and external resources (components C and E) also serve to either buffer or worsen the impact of health problems on older adults' quality of life. As our case studies illustrated, both Tom and Marge engaged in proactive adaptations to enhance their lives. Tom had the financial resources (an important external resource) to help him maintain his quality of life by allowing him to travel and to engage in regular social activities, including eating out with friends and participating in golf outings. On the other hand, Marge had financial problems throughout the course of the study and reported that her finances sometimes limited her ability to purchase what she needed. Marge is an excellent example of how a person with poor financial resources can work toward successful aging. When she was no longer able to exercise, she substituted the time she devoted to exercising with her favorite hobby—knitting—and found great meaning in making items to give to loved ones as well as to strangers.

We also want to briefly highlight how social institutions can hinder or facilitate proactive adaptations. At best, they empower older people (Thursz et al., 1995), while at worst they can contribute to learned helplessness (Baltes, 1995). Legal and policy initiatives can serve to facilitate or place constraints on proactivity. We will proceed to illustrate these influences in selected areas of proactivity. In considering policy and legal influences, it is useful to distinguish their intent from their implementation. Many laws are intended to protect frail and vulnerable aged populations, such as those with dementia, or those living in institutional settings. Yet, implementation of these protections often poses problems for continued autonomy or self expression of the vulnerable group they aim to serve, which are key underpinnings of proactivity.

The following examples highlight how legal or policy initiatives may facilitate or hinder diverse forms of proactivity.

Role Substitution. To the extent that older adults may wish to enter or return to work roles after social losses, such as becoming widowed, legal protection can serve important preventive functions. Age discrimination laws in the United States can protect older workers from job loss, enabling them to continue gainful employment. Once again, however, legal protection enters only in extreme cases where damage may have already occurred and subtle forms of age discrimination in hiring and layoffs have been well documented. In the United State, Social Security reforms in 2000 have removed penalties to wage earners who receive Social Security giving older persons greater freedom to supplement postretirement income by continued work engagement.

Environmental Modifications. The Americans with Disabilities Act has resulted in mandated environmental modifications in public buildings (e.g., adapting curbsides for wheelchair use). Although this law has been slow in implementation, it is now more possible for disabled older adults to be able to attend movies, lectures, and classes. This law has generally made it easier for older adults with disabilities to continue to conduct day-to-day activities. In addition, access to transportation has been increased as both public and private transportation companies are now required to provide services to disabled older adults. It is also notable that some communities such as Dunedin, Florida, actively cater to older residents by environmental modifications, such as increasing the length of green lights to facilitate crossing streets for older pedestrians. These are examples in which policies and legal protections serve to facilitate continued late life proactivity.

Health Care Consumerism. Health care consumerism is an important emergent form of proactivity among older adults. This is a very complex area wherein laws have conflicting consequences for patients. In the United States, laws are increasingly protecting patients' rights to view and obtain medical records. Having accurate information about one's diagnosis and treatments are a cornerstone for taking proactive actions and engaging in advocacy. Nevertheless, while these laws are on the books, medical institutions have been resistant in implementing release of information to patients (Kahana & Kahana, 2001).

Other important aspects of legal protection for patients relates to the right to refuse treatment and to provide advanced directives for end-of-life care. Here again, the intentions are good, but control is often illusory. Thus, for example, in nursing homes and hospitals, elderly patients are required to be informed about their right to provide directives about end-of-life decisions. Yet, the language of these documents is so arcane and full of legal jargon that many patients feel threatened and unsure of what they are signing. Further, the legal concerns of physicians and health care institutions about possible lawsuits have represented a problematic situation for health care consumerism because of the consequent common practice of defensive medicine.

Technology Use. One of the key deterrents for use of technology in the form of assistive devices is their cost. Medicare has historically been very slow to cover new technologies. Steps are currently being taken to speed up this process, but the burden of proof of need for a new technology still lies on the shoulders of the elderly individual using it (Tunis & Kang, 2001).

Use of electronic patient records allows all physicians caring for an individual (primary care doctor as well as specialist) to immediately view and add entries to a current chart (Safran, Sands, & Rind, 1999). Allowing patients to e-mail their physicians improves care because e-mails are less likely to be lost than are transcribed phone messages, and, for noncritical needs, communication through e-mail ensures that patients and doctors do not waste time on an unneeded office visit (Sands, 1999). Nevertheless, physicians have been slow to embrace such technology, potentially because of fears of sharing control or power with patients.

CONCLUSION

This chapter aimed to provide some examples of the ways in which older adults' proactive adaptations can help facilitate maintenance of high quality of life and consequently successful aging even in the face of chronic illness. Older adults value independence and seek to maintain autonomy even when ill health curtails their engagement in strenuous work or leisure pursuits. Our model of successful aging points to processes of proactive adaptations whereby the negative effects of illness-related stressors on well-being may be ameliorated. We also maintain that even when positive outcomes of well-being cannot be attained in the face of chronic illness, the human agency, effort, and striving inherent in proactive adaptations may signify successful aging. Our discussion is also aimed to empower older people, who will, in increasing numbers, face the challenges of chronic illness to take their rightful place at the table of those judged by society as aging successfully. Awareness of policy makers, service professionals, and gerontological scholars of options for potential of the chronically ill aged to adapt effectively can help in the process of such empowerment, particularly through removing institutional obstacles and reinforcing individual initiatives toward proactive adaptations.

REFERENCES

The American Health Assistance Foundation. (2002). *Heart disease and stroke risk factors.* Retrieved from http://www.ahaf.org/hrtsrok/about/hsrisk_body.htm.

Antonucci, T. C., & Akiyama, H. (1991). Social relationships and aging well. *Generations, 15*(1), 39–44.

The Arthritis Foundation. (2002). Retrieved from www.arthritis.org/.

Baltes, M. M. (1995). Dependency in old age: Gains and losses. *Current Directions in Psychological Science, 4*(1), 14–19.

Bettermann, H., von Bonin, D., Fruhwirth, M., Cysarz, D., & Moser, M. (2002). Effects of speech therapy with poetry on heart rate rhythmicity and cardiorespiratory coordination. *International Journal of Cardiology, 84*(1), 77–88.

Borawski, E., Kinney, J., & Kahana, E. (1996). The meaning of older adults' health appraisals: Congruence with health status and determinants of mortality. *Journal of Gerontology, 51B*(3), S157–S170.

Boult, C., Kane, R. L., Louis, T. A., Boult, L., & McCaffrey, D. (1994). Chronic conditions that lead to functional limitation in the elderly. *Journal of Gerontology, 49*(10), M28–M36.

Bradley C., & Speight J. (2002). Patient perceptions of diabetes and diabetes therapy: Assessing quality of life. *Diabetes Metabolic Research Review, 18*(3), S64–S69.

Burckhardt, C. S. (1988). Quality of life for women with arthritis. *Health Care for Women International, 9*(4), 229–235.

Cantor, M. H. (1979). The informal support system in New York's inner city elderly: Is ethnicity a factor? In D. E. Gefland & A. J. Kutznik (Eds.), *Ethnicity and aging* (pp. 153–174). New York: Springer Publishing.

Carstensen, L. L., & Freud, A. M. (1994). The resilience of the aging self. *Developmental Review, 14*(1), 81–92.

Desai, M. M., Zhang, P., & Hennessy, C. H. (1999). Surveillance for morbidity and mortality among older adults—United States, 1995–1996. *Morbidity and Mortality Weekly Report, 48*(8), 7–25.

Downe-Wamboldt, B. L., & Melanson, P. M. (1998). A causal model of coping and well-being in elderly people with arthritis. *Journal of Advanced Nursing, 27*(6), 1109–1116.

Gallo, J. J., Rebok, G. W., & Lesikar, S. E. (1999). Driving habits of adults aged 60 years and older. *Journal of the American Geriatrics Society, 47*(3), 335–341.

Guerette, P., Nakai, R., Verran, A., & Sommerville, N. (1992). *Safety begins at home: A practical guide for professionals, older adults, and their families.* Downey, CA: Rehabilitation Research & Training Center on Aging, Rancho Los Amigos Medical Center, University of Southern California.

Hagestad, G. O., & Dannefer, D. (2001). Concepts and theories of aging: Beyond microfication in social science approaches. In R. H. Binstock & L. K. George (Eds.), *Handbook of aging and the social sciences* (pp. 3–21). San Diego: Academic Press.

Horstman, J. (1999, March–April). Movement therapies. *Arthritis Today.* Retrieved from http://www.arthritis.org/resources/arthritistoday/Default.asp

Hurley B. F., & Roth S. M. (2000). Strength training in the elderly: Effects on risk factors for age-related diseases. *Sports Medicine, 30*(4), 249–268.

Jette, A. M. (1996). Disability trends and transitions. In R. H. Binstock & L. K. George (Eds.), *Handbook of aging and the social sciences* (4th ed., pp. 94–116). San Diego: Academic Press.

Kaboli, P. J., Doebbeling, B. N., Saag, K. G., & Rosenthal, G. E. (2001). Use of complementary and alternative medicine by older patients with arthritis: A population-based study. *Arthritis and Rheumatism, 45*(4), 398–403.

Kahana, E., & Borawski, E. (1997). Altruism and helping others as proactive adaptations in late life: How helping others returns dividends. *Gerontologist, 1*(37), 290.

Kahana, E., Chirayath, H. T., Wisniewski, A., Kahana, B., & Kercher, K. (2003). *The role of health-related adaptations in ameliorating adverse effects of ill health on quality of life of the aged.* Paper to be presented at the 2003 meeting of the American Sociological Association. Atlanta, GA.

Kahana, E., & Kahana, B. (1996). Conceptual and empirical advances in understanding aging well through proactive adaptation. In V. Bengtson (Ed.), *Adulthood and aging: Research on continuities and discontinuities* (pp. 18–41). New York: Springer Publishing.

Kahana, E., & Kahana, B. (2001). On being a proactive health care consumer: Making an "unresponsive" system work for you. *Research in Sociology of Health Care: Changing Consumers and Changing Technology in Health Care and Health Care Delivery, 19,* 21–44.

Kahana, E., & Kahana, B. (2003). Contextualizing successful aging: New directions in age-old search. In R. Settersten, Jr. (Ed.), *Invitation to the life course: A new look at old age* (pp. 225–255). Amityville, NY: Baywood Publishing.

Kahana, E., Kahana, B., & Deimling, G. (in press). Patient proactivity enhancing doctor-patient-family communication in cancer prevention and care among the aged. *Journal of Patient Education and Counseling.*

Kahana, E., Kahana, B, & Kercher, K. (in press). Emerging lifestyles and proactive options for successful aging. *Ageing International.*

Kahana, E., King, C., Brown, J., DeCrane, P., Mackey, D., Monaghan, et al. (1994). Environmental modifications and disabled elders. In J. C. Rey & C. Tilquin (Eds.), *Proceedings of the fifth international conference on systems sciences in health-social services for the elderly and the disabled* (pp. 145–150). Montréal: Science des Systemes

Kahana, E., Lawrence, R.H., Kahana, B., Kercher, K., Wisniewski, A., Stoller, E., et al. (2002). Long-term impact of preventive proactivity on quality of life of the old-old. *Psychosomatic Medicine, 64*(3), 382–394.

Lawhon, T., & Ennis, D. (1995). Technology impacts older Americans. *Activities, Adaptation and Aging, 20*(2), 51–64.

Lawton, M. P. (1990). Residential environment and self-directedness among older people. *American Psychologist, 45*(5), 638–640.

Lee, S., O'Neill, G., & Summer, L. (2000). Heart disease: A disabling yet preventable condition. *Challenges for the 21st century: Chronic and disabling conditions, 3,* 1–6.

Liebl, A. (2002). Challenges in optimal metabolic control of diabetes. *Diabetes Metabolic Research Review, 18*(3), S36–41.

Link, B. G., & Phelan, J. (1995). Social conditions as fundamental causes of disease. *Journal of Health and Social Behavior,* 80–94.

Mann, W. C., Hurren, D., & Tomita, M. (1995). Assistive devices used by home-based elderly persons with arthritis. *American Journal of Occupational Therapy, 49*(8), 810–820.

Mazzeo R. S., & Tanaka, H. (2001). Exercise prescription for the elderly: Current recommendations. *Sports Medicine, 31*(11), 809–818.

McGowin, D. F. (1993). *Living in the labyrinth: A personal journey through the maze of Alzheimer's.* San Francisco: ElderBooks.

Meneilly, G. S., & Tessier, D. (2001). Diabetes in elderly adults. *Journals of Gerontology—Biological Sciences and Medical Sciences, 56*(1), M5–M13.

Menne, H. L., Kinney, J. M., & Morhardt, D. J. (2002). Trying to continue to do as much as they can do': Theoretical insights regarding continuity and meaning making in the face of dementia. *Dementia: The International Journal of Social Research and Practice, 1*(3), 367–382.

Miller, T. D., Balady, G. J., & Fletcher, G. F. (1997). Exercise and its role in the prevention and rehabilitation of cardiovascular disease. *Annals of Behavioral Medicine, 19*(3), 220–229.

National Academy on an Aging Society. (1999, November). *Chronic conditions. A challenge for the 21st century.* Washington, DC: National Academy on an Aging Society.

The National Academy on an Aging Society. (2000). *Heart disease: A disabling yet preventable condition.* Retrieved from http://www.agingsociety.org

National Center for Chronic Disease Prevention and Health Promotion. (2002). *Healthy aging.* Washington, DC: Center for Disease Control. Retrieved from www.cdc.gov/

Nordenskiold, U. (1997). Daily activities in women with rheumatoid arthritis: Aspects of patient education, assistive devices and methods for disability and impairment assessment. *Scandinavian Journal of Rehabilitation Medicine Supplement, 37,* 1–72.

Panusch, R. S., & Holtz, H. A. (1994). Is exercise good or bad for arthritis in the elderly? *Southern Medical Journal, 87*(5), S74–79.

Pasanisi F., Contaldo F., de Simone, G., & Mancini, M. (2001). Benefits of sustained moderate weight loss in obesity. *Nutrition Metabolic Cardiovascular Disease, 11*(6), 401–406.

Pearlin, L., Lieberman, M., Menaghan, E., & Mullan, J. (1981). The stress process. *Journal of Health and Social Behavior, 22*(4), 337–356.

Pennebacker, J. (Ed.). (1995). *Emotion disclosure and health.* Washington, DC: American Psychological Association.

Post, S. G., & Whitehouse, P. J. (1995). *Fairhill guidelines on ethics of the care of people with Alzheimer's disease: A clinical summary.* Cleveland, OH: Case Western Reserve University.

Robert Wood Johnson Foundation. (1996). *Chronic care in America: A 21st century challenge.* Princeton, NJ: Robert Wood Johnson Foundation.

Rodwin, M. A. (1997). The neglected remedy: Strengthening consumer voice in managed care. *The American Prospect, 8*(34), 45–50.

Rogers, P. J. (2001). A healthy body, a healthy mind: Long-term impact of diet on mood and cognitive function. *Proceedings of the Nutrition Society, 60*(1), 135–143.

Rowe, J., & Kahn R. (1998). *Successful aging.* New York: Pantheon.

Safran, C., Sands, D. Z., & Rind, D. M. (1999). Online medical records: A decade of experience. *Methods of Information Medicine, 38*(4/5), 308–312.

Sands, D. Z. (1999). Electronic patient-centered communication: Managing risks, managing opportunities, managing care. *American Journal of Managed Care, 5*(12), 1569–1571.

Settersten, R. (2003). *Invitation to the life course: A new look at old age* (pp. 225–255). Amityville, NY: Baywood Publishing.

Shirey, L., & Summer, L. (2000). At risk: Developing chronic conditions later in life. *Challenges for the 21st Century: Chronic and Disabling Conditions, 4,* 1–6.

Skoog, I., Blennow, K., & Marcusson, J. (1996). Dementia. In J. E. Birren (Ed.), *Encyclopedia of gerontology* (Vol. 1, pp. 383–403). San Diego: Academic Press, Inc.

Starren, J., Hripcsak, G., Sengupta, S., Abbruscato, C. R., Knudson, P. E., Weinstock, R. S., et al. (2002). Columbia University's informatics for diabetes education and telemedicine (IDEATel) project: Technical implementation. *Journal of the American Medical Informatics Association, 9*(1), 25–36.

Tabbarah, M., Silverstein, M., & Seeman, T. (2000). A health and demographic profile of noninstitutionalized older Americans residing in environments with home modifications. *Journal of Aging and Health, 12*(2), 204–228.

Thursz, D., Nusberg, C., & Prather, J. (1995). *Empowering older people.* Westport, CT: Auburn House.

Tunis, S. R., & Kang, J. L. (2001). Improvements in Medicare coverage of new technology. *Health Affairs, 20*(5), 83–85.

White, H., McConnell, E., Clipp, E., Bynum, L., Teague, C., Navas, L., et al. (1999). Surfing the Net in later life: A review of the literature and pilot study of computer use and quality of life. *Journal of Applied Gerontology, 18*(3), 358–378.

Winters, C. A. (1997). Living with chronic heart disease: A pilot study. *The Qualitative Report, 3*(4). Retrieved from http://www.nova.edu/ssss/QR/QR3-4/winters.html

PART III

Aging Across Generations— Interactions That Work

Peter J. Whitehouse

This concluding section of the book has four chapters written from a variety of different disciplinary perspectives, including medicine, nursing, psychology, gerontology and social work. The authors focus on the importance of families in providing care for older adults, particularly the role of women. The particular challenges for grandparent caregivers of children are identified as well as the importance of developing programs targeted for those individuals. In addition to describing the challenges that intergenerational caregiving presents, the authors also communicate a sense of caring and hope about the positive growth opportunities for individuals and families through this process.

The first chapter begins with a clinical story of a devoted daughter who tries to provide a good quality of life for a moderately demented and medically frail mother. The circumstances of her death are less than ideal and highlight the importance of communication between professional and family caregivers. This first chapter presents the idea that the very structures of our families are changing creating an enormous amount of variability that health care professionals need to address as they attend to the needs of caregivers. This chapter by Peter DeGolia is written from a family medicine perspective and offers very practical advice about how caregivers should address the challenges of caregiving, including taking care of themselves, recognizing limits and developing regular planned schedules of activities. He ends the chapter by discussing a variety of sources of support for the caregiver, yet realizing that family and friends often remain their best source of assistance.

The next chapter by Carol Musil and colleagues begins with the theme of caregiving from a family perspective and includes aspects of gender and ethnicity. They point out that the concept of "bread winner" for women is a relatively modern one and although the roles of women have changed through time, the focus on home and care remains consistent. The article states that as women assume more responsibilities in the professional realm, dramatic effects on their abilities to provide satisfactory care at home have occurred. These authors highlight the emerging role of grandparents as primary caregivers. Almost four million grandparents are raising grandchildren in this country, most of whom are grandmothers. The importance of building intergenerational ties, particularly through ethnic bonds is emphasized in the chapter. A common heritage, history and geography of shared ethnic backgrounds can be a source of support both conceptually and practically to caregivers.

The next chapter by Cameron Camp and colleagues describes evaluating a program for clients with dementia; a topic referred to in the background of earlier chapters is brought to the fore. The presence of cognitive impairment in a care recipient adds to the caregiving challenges. This chapter presents a study on the effects of intergenerational relationships on families. In this particular study the authors worked with individuals who had cognitive impairment and offered them the opportunity to mentor young children. They describe previous work that has shown intergenerational programming to increase levels of social interaction in adult day care. Their carefully designed studies include a variety of measures to determine the impact of these care relationships on the people affected with dementia. As in previous studies they use Montessori based activities that have been found to be appropriate for both the older adults with cognitive impairment and children. Over an extended period of time they used a variety of measures to assess the impact of this intervention on the adults, including instrument such as their own Myers Research Institute Engagement Scale and Ratings of Affect. They compared the scores of participants in the mentoring program to the children with participants in regularly scheduled day care activities. Importantly, they did find that there were short-term benefits of seniors interacting with children, even though these effects did not persist after the study.

The final chapter of this section focuses on the broader conceptions of intergenerational health and a series of programs developed in an innovative community organization: Fairhill Center. The major focus of this chapter is on the world's first public intergenerational school in which a variety of programs have been developed to promote shared learning experiences between older adults and kindergarten through fourth graders. Like previous chapters, this section stresses the importance of future intergenerational health issues. They highlight the importance of developing partnerships between educational organizations and long-term care providers. They describe further a variety of programs in the Intergenerational School in which children and older adults have shared stories and other activities. Programs with undergraduate students at Case Western Reserve University reflect the idea that intergenerational programs do not have to involve just the very young and very old. Thus individuals of many different ages can come together to share learning experiences.

Chapters in this section highlight the importance of families and communities taking creative and imaginative approaches to providing care across the generations. Whether it is in a doctor's office, nurse's clinic, school classroom or long-term care facility, the value of intergenerational learning and care can be realized. With such a positive outlook, the challenges of an increasing aged population will be more easily addressed and overcome.

CHAPTER 7

Multigenerational Issues That Impact on Successful Aging in Seniors: Caregiving—A Precious Gift

Peter A. DeGolia

In any family in which there is an individual with an acute and life-threatening or chronic and long-term illness or disease, the caregiver is under considerable stress (Medalie et al., 2002).

—Jack Medalie, MD
Professor Emeritus
Department of Family Medicine
Case Western Reserve University
School of Medicine

Let me out of this hotel prison!

—Jane Doe
97-year-old woman
Resident of an Assisted Living Facility

Jane Doe was 97 years of age when she died, most probably from an acute pulmonary embolism associated with prolonged immobilization following a course of influenza. Her daughter Janie was 74 at the time of her death. Jane had 2 children, 7 grandchildren, and 9 great grandchildren at the time of her passing.

Jane had mild to moderate dementia (not formally diagnosed), hypertension, and osteoporosis. She was hard-headed and quite set in her ways. For her entire adult life, she relied heavily on the companionship and interaction of her daughter. Their two lives were very closely intertwined—common friends, common social organizations, similar activities and interests. As Jane aged, her independence became more limited. Traumatic and difficult events, such as two car accidents resulting in the revocation of driver's license, forgetting to pay financial bills, and increasing need for assistance in daily activities resulted in her transfer to an assisted living facility (ALF). With each event—and as her functional status declined—tension increased between her and her daughter. By default, Jane's daughter was the primary decision-maker. Jane's son offered financial support and cameo appearances, but did not offer to do any of the "heavy lifting"—such as listening to his mother's concerns or transporting her to the grocery store, clothing stores, or the hair dresser. Jane was prone to histrionic outbursts. She successfully played each sibling off the other, but at a high price.

Janie suffered from excessive guilt mixed with great frustration. Anger was a common expression, irritability ever present. She was depressed and suffered from insomnia. Her relationship with her brother suffered irreparable damage. Janie's relationship with her husband and her children suffered as well.

Care for her mother was always a top priority for Janie. Two years before her mother's death, Janie moved 60 miles away to a new home. She continued to commute frequently to care for her mother. When her mother could no longer live safely on her own, Janie arranged to move her mother into a continuing care retirement community (CCRC) assisted living apartment within 5 minutes of her home. Jane hated the "hotel prison," as she called it, and castigated her daughter unmercifully for placing her in that institution. Although she adapted well to her new environment and, after several difficult months, even began to interact with others and participate in limited social activities, she never forgave her daughter for taking away her independence. Janie's guilt never resolved, even though she knew her mother was safe, well cared for, and living close by.

Jane contacted influenza and was transferred to the CCRC's skilled nursing facility. Her care was inadequate, and she was left in bed long after she began to recover. One afternoon, Jane developed acute respiratory distress, tachypnea, and extreme anxiety. Not having completed advance directives, and instead of responding to the emergent situation, the nursing staff called her daughter for guidance. Janie, however, was exhausted, preoccupied with personal affairs, and unable to cope with the situation as presented by the nursing staff. When she received the telephone call from the nurse, her first impression was that her mother was being histrionic and acting out because Janie had not visited recently. Not being a medical person, Janie was not able to fully consider the clinical implications of her mother's condition as presented by the nursing staff. Janie instructed the nursing staff to contact the facility physician for an anxiolytic medication. Jane died in the nurse's arms, frightened and feeling abandoned, an hour later.

CAREGIVING AND SUCCESSFUL AGING

Successful aging depends, in part, on successful community and family systems of care. As people age, chronic diseases accumulate that can negatively impact our ability to live independently in the community of our choosing. Caregivers and community systems of care enable many older persons to continue to live successful lives outside of institutions. Caregiving often effects multiple generations. Caring for an ill and debilitated loved one or friend is common in the United States today. Approximately 52 million Americans care for a family member with mental or physical impairment (Survey, US HHS, 1999). As our society ages, this number can be expected to continue to increase. It is estimated that the population over 65 years of age will double in the next 30 years. The fastest growing segment of our society is the age cohort consisting of those who are 85 years old or older (Gilford, 1988).

Chronic disease management has become the primary focus of medical encounters involving older persons. With aging comes an increase in the incidence and prevalence of chronic diseases. These diseases, depending on type and severity, can result in increased dependency upon other people for activities related to daily living (Elston et al., 1991). Studies have shown that family support of an impaired or chronically ill member affects the outcome of the chronic medical illness (Campbell & McDaniel, 2001).

Who becomes the caregiver usually depends on the gender of the patient. The majority of caregivers are older women—wives, daughters, or daughter-in-laws (Biegel et al., 1991). Women have a longer life expectancy and often outlive their husbands. Older men often have spouses who care for them, while older women rely on a daughter or daughter-in-law. Population data show that men tend to marry younger women. When their spouses do die, they tend to remarry. Women whose spouses die generally do not remarry (Gilford, 1998). The spouse-spouse relationship is different from the parent-child relationship (Able, 1987).

Family members continue to provide the vast majority of assistance to dependent older persons (Haley, 1997). The degree of assistance varies with the type and severity of the patient's dependency. The important common tasks provided by caregivers include the following:

1. To provide health care professionals with accurate medical information. This includes past medical history as well as onset, duration, and severity of active symptoms.
2. To manage the ongoing needs of the dependent person, which can include arranging medical visits, coordinating and providing transportation, and supervising the adherence of prescribed medical and pharmaceutical regimens.
3. To perform personal care tasks and household chores such as laundry, shopping, and housecleaning. These may be the most demanding activity experienced by caregivers.
4. To do advance care planning. This task is often overlooked. Communicating with the dependent older person about their health care values and goals, discussing advance directives, future medical and housing needs, and being called upon to make health care decisions as a proxy are difficult and stress-provoking responsibilities (Silliman, 2000).

ROLE OF THE HEALTH PROVIDER IN ASSESSING CAREGIVER STRESS

Caregiver burden has been studied by Zarit (Zarit et al., 1980) and described as encompassing the physical, emotional, and financial toll associated with providing care to a dependent person (Geroge et al., 1986). The degree of behavioral problems in patients with dementia has been shown to contribute to caregiver burden (Baumgarten et al., 1994). Caregiver skills have been shown to correlate with caregiver burden. Coping skills and management strategies lower levels of burden (Saad et al., 1995).

The primary medical provider who has worked with the patient from initial evaluation through diagnosis and treatment can be instrumental in identifying caregiver stress and providing needed assistance to the caregiver to help optimize patient care (Dunkin & Anderson-Hanley, 1998). This is especially helpful for patients new to a provider's practice or those presenting a situation that is beyond the usual scope of practice of the provider. A Comprehensive geriatric assessment can be a valuable tool to help primary care providers and caregivers assess the special needs of the older patient. This type of assessment medical service uses a team approach to evaluate a person with chronic, complex medical problems. Part of the evaluation should include assessment of caregiver status and needs. Caregiver burden can be assessed systematically by focusing on areas of mental health, social support, resources, and coping skills. Parks developed a screening questionnaire that can be used in an office-based setting to review these areas of concern (Parks et al., 2000). Mental health questions should focus on a person feeling under stress, depressed, and anxious. Social support questions should identify contact with other family members and friends through visits or telephone calls. Asking if a caregiver has outside sources of help explores issues of resource support. Coping skills can be explored by asking what a caregiver does to relieve stress and tension.

The health care provider should be aware of outside resources that may be of assistance to a caregiver. A wide variety of resources are available to caregivers; these are listed later. A relatively new development is the availability of advance practice nurses and social workers with skills in life care planning for older adults and distant family members. These health professionals provide guidance and help to coordinate care for elders in need of the assistance. This is thought to be particularly useful for distant family members who cannot provide ongoing onsite coordination of care (Haley, 1997). Adult day care centers, respite care services, agencies providing meals on wheels, and local nursing agencies providing personal care services are important resources available to caregivers. Adult day services are generally well received by families and can delay institutionalization (Lawton et al., 1989). These programs serve as a form of respite care. It is not unusual for the health care professional to give the caregiver permission to use respite services.

Coping strategies can be emotion-focused or problem-focused. A problem-focused response would involve stating a specific strategy for addressing the problem, such as contacting the nurse for assistance in understanding what is taking place. Emotion-focused responses to challenging problems should be seen as a red flag to potential caregiver stress. These responses are stated in terms of one's feelings, such as crying or anger. Constructing a larger sense of the illness has been shown to have a lower incidence of depression among caregivers (Saad et al., 1995).

Another important role of the health care provider is to disseminate health information. A lack of understanding by the caregiver and family about a person's disease process may increase caregiver stress. The caregiver's knowledge about the disease process and available resources should be explored. Provider education often includes basic information about the disease process as experienced by the impaired adult. Providing insight as to disease trajectory and what can be expected as the disease progresses is also very important. Anticipatory guidance to family members as to what may be expected of them is often necessary.

Finally, a health care provider should be monitoring for special conditions that are either highly associated with increased caregiver stress or are prone to problematic outcomes. Cognitively impaired elders present a special challenge. The literature is abundant regarding issues of care and stress associated with this population. It has been shown that caregivers of persons with a dementing illness spend an average of 60 hours per week providing care at home, over a median time span of 6.5 years (Max et al., 1995). Elder abuse and neglect is another area of concern and when signs are present they represent to the care provider red flags for caregiver stress (McGuire & Fulmer, 1997). Physical signs including bruises, burns, or malnutrition are often most easily identified. Emotional and financial abuse is more difficult to assess. Screening questions such as "Has anyone at home ever hurt you?", "Has anyone taken anything that was yours without asking?", and "Have you ever signed any document that you did not understand?" can be asked to begin to explore this possibility (Silliman, 2000).

Advance care planning and identification of the older patient's desires for end-of-life care is an important part of the on-going discussion between a health care provider and the person for whom they are caring. The patient's proxy decision-maker and family members should be involved in this discussion. Their engagement is essential if the dependent person does not have the capacity for self-care decision- making. Failure to not have these discussions can lead to heightened tension for the caregiver, family, and health professional staff as an end-of-life situation evolves.

CONSEQUENCES OF CAREGIVING

Caregiving is a demanding job. It can be a life-threatening activity as well (Schulz, 1999). Many caregivers feel inadequate in their ability to meet the needs of the person for whom they are caring. Associated with this commitment are emotional hurdles that significantly increase the burden of care for the caregiver. Frustration and guilt are commonly experienced by caregivers. Frustration often results from a caregiver feeling he or she cannot do everything that is desired by the person. Guilt is a consequence of recognizing the inability to do everything and believing that the person is not being provided the level of service needed. This is a pervasive and destructive emotion, which is often expressed as retrospective criticism of what could have been done better, more completely, or differently to have changed a clinical outcome. Anger and resentment are other emotional hurdles faced by caregivers. An Indiana University study of 3,000 caregivers found the longer one cared for a loved one, the more likely one was to suffer depression, insomnia, and even physical problems (*Journal of Health and Social Behavior,* 2000).

Grief and a feeling of extreme sadness is another burden felt by caregivers. It is an extraordinary individual who can care for one's loved one and simultaneously face the reality that one will lose that person. When caring for a terminally ill person, the end of this person's life is often anticipated but desperately avoided.

The group of individuals involved in taking care of the everyday affairs of the patient and family is known as the functional family. In any family in which there is an individual with an acute and life-threatening or chronic and long-term illness or diseases, the caregiver is under considerable stress. Unless the caregiver receives sufficient support from the family and/or others, coping mechanisms will fail and the caregiver will develop overt or covert signs of illness (Campbell & McDaniel, 2001).

COPING STRATEGIES FOR PREVENTING CAREGIVER BURNOUT

It is important to recognize signs of caregiver stress and burnout. These include complaints of feeling stress and exhaustion as well as depression and anxiety. Other common signs include irritability, insomnia, and the deterioration of relationships with other people. In addition to the personal toll on the caregiver, caregiver stress that is allowed to fester unchecked can have detrimental effects for the patient. Patient neglect, including bedsores, weight loss, and dehydration, can result (Schulz, 1995).

Preventive steps should be taken to limit the guilt, frustration, and grief one can experience as a caregiver. By reducing the stress experienced by the caregiver, the ability of the caregiver to be able to continue to provide the necessary service can be extended. Clarifying with the patient and/or decision maker the type of care that is desired can help alleviate feelings of guilt and frustration. For example, does the person want to live alone?; Can the person live alone?; Does the person want or need assistance with activities of daily living?; Are there sufficient financial resources to augment the level of care desired by the person?; and, How much time does the caregiver need to devote to caregiving? Caregivers need attention, too. It is important for health care providers to support caregivers and help them understand they are not alone.

There are seven important steps caregivers should take to avoid burnout (Caregiver's Cycle of Guilt)

1. Acknowledge limitations. This is often a difficult step for many caregivers. It can be a major source of guilt. Recognition that each one of us has limitations as to what we can and cannot do, as well as a basic need to preserve our own physical and emotional health, can be a serious step toward preserving one's ability to be an effective caregiver.
2. Prioritize daily tasks. Identify what must be done for that day and what can be accomplished.
3. Plan regular respites from caregiving. Work out a schedule where time is preserved for meeting personal needs and activities. Making time for exercise, eating properly, and getting adequate rest are essential activities for every caregiver.
4. Give permission to be imperfect. It is important for the caregiver to focus on the good they are doing for the dependent person.
5. Become educated about the disease of the person for whom care is being provided.

6. Ask for help. Recognize that there are resources in each community that can assist in the task of caregiving. Caregivers should be encouraged to seek assistance from family; neighbors; church, synagogue, or mosque; workplace; and formal and informal caregivers.
   a. Identify organizations, such as the Alzheimer's Association, that have support groups that can educate and empower caregivers.
7. Accept emotional support from family and friends.

While the emotional burdens associated with caregiving can be substantial, the benefits are tremendous. Caregivers often develop empathy for the care recipient and for other caregivers. Caregiving promotes an awareness of the physical and emotional trials and tribulations experienced by others in similar situations. Perhaps the most important aspect of caregiving is the expression of compassionate love. Caregiving provides the opportunity for one person to assist another person in a direct and tangible way. The act of caring and providing assistance to another person is a precious gift. The act of caregiving can enhance self-worth and promote a sense of accomplishment.

SOURCES OF POTENTIAL SUPPORT
FOR THE CAREGIVER

Informal caregiving resources
Family
Neighbors
Church, synagogue, or mosque
The workplace

Formal caregiving resources
Social Service Agencies
Personal care aides
Chore services
Senior Companion
Senior day care programs
Meals on Wheels
Nursing Care Agencies

Skilled nursing
Private duty
Personal care
Program for All inclusive Care for the Elderly (PACE) (local programs in 26 cities across the United States)
EverCare Connections (nationwide fee-for-service eldercare referral and evaluation program)

Secondary Caregiver Services
Home Durable Medical Equipment Companies
Transportation and Delivery services

Advocacy agencies
Area Agency on Aging
City, State, or County Agency on Aging
Alzheimer's Association

Other sources
Your primary care physician
Life Care Advisor
Legal Services
    Adult Protective Services
    Guardianship

RESOURCES FOR OBTAINING INFORMATION ABOUT CARE GIVING

Alzheimer's Association
    800-272-3900
    www.alzheimers.org

American Association of Retired Persons (AARP)
    800-424-3410

Children of Aging Parents
    800-227-7294
    www.careguide.cgi/caps/capshome.htm

National Family Caregivers Association
    800-896-3650
    www.nfcacares.org

Eldercare Locator
  800-677-1116

Caregiving Online
  www.caregiving.com

CareGuide.com
  www.careguide.com

Caregiverzone.com
  www.caregiverzone.com

REFERENCES

Able, E. K (1987). *Love is not enough: Family care of the frail elderly.* Washington, DC: American Public Health Association.

Adelman, R., Greene, M., & Ory, M. (2000). Communication between older patients and their physicians. *Clinics in Geriatric Medicine, 16*(1), 1–24.

Baumgarten, M., Hanley, J., Infante-Rivard, C., Battista, R., Becker, R., & Gauthier, S. (1994). Health of family members caring for elderly persons with dementia. *Annals of Internal Medicine, 120*(2), 126–132.

Biegel, D. E., Sales, E., & Schulz, R. (1991). *Family care giving in chronic illness: Alzheimer's disease, cancer, heart disease, mental illness, and stroke.* Newbury Park, CA: Sage.

Campbel, T. L., & McDaniel, S. H. (2001). Behavioral medicine in family practice. *Clinicas in Family Practice, 3*(1).

Caregiver's Cycle of Guilt. Retrieved from www.carescot.com/resources/caregiver/cycle_of_guilt.htm

Dunkin, J. J., & Anderson-Hanley, C. (1998). Dementia caregiver burden: A review of the literature and guidelines for assessment and intervention. *Neurology, 51*(1, Suppl. 1), S53–60.

Elston, J., Koch, G. G., & Weissert, W. G. (1991). Regression-adjusted small area estimates of functional dependency in the non-institutionalized American population age 65 and over. *American Journal of Public Health, 81*(3), 355–339.

Freedman, V. A,, & Martin, L. G. (1998). Understanding trends in functional limitations among older Americans. *American Journal of Public Health, 88*(10), 1457–1462.

George, L., & Gwyther, L. (1986). Caregiver well-being: A multidimensional examination of family caregivers of demented adults. *Gerontologist, 26*(3), 253–259.

Gilford, D. M (Ed.). (1988). *The aging population in the twenty-first century: Statistics for health policy.* Washington, DC: National Academy Press.

Haley, W. E. (1997). The family caregiver's role in Alzheimer's disease: *Neurology, 48*(Suppl. 6), S25–29.

Lawton, M., Brody, E., & Saperstein, A. (1989). A controlled study of respite service for caregivers of Alzheimer's patients. *Gerontologist, 29*(1), 8–16.

Max, W., Webber, P., & Fox, P. (1995). Alzheimer's disease: The unpaid burden of caring. *Journal of Aging Health, 7,* 179.

Medalie, J. H., & Cole-Kelly, K. (2002, April). The clinical importance of defining family. *American Family Physician, 65*(7), 1277.

McGuire, P., & Fulmer, T. (1997). Elder abuse. In C. K. Cassel et al., (Ed.), *Geriatric Medicine* (3rd ed., pp.855–864). New York: Springer-Verlag.

Parks, S. M., & Novielli, K. (2000). A practical guide to caring for caregivers. *American Family Physician, 62*(12), 2613–2620.

Saad, K., Hartman, J., Ballard, C., Kurian, M., Graham, C., & Wilcock, G. (1995). Coping by the carers of dementia sufferers. *Age Aging, 24*(6), 495–498.

Schultz, R., Brien, A., Bookwala, J., & Fleissner, K. (1995). Psychiatric and physical effects of Alzheimer's disease caregiving: Prevalence, correlates, and causes. *Gerontologist, 35*(6), 771–791.

Schulz, R., & Beach, S. (1999). Care giving as a risk factor for mortality: The care giver health effects study. *Journal of the American Medical Association, 282*(23), 2215–2219.

Survey, US HHS, 1999.

Zarit, S. H., Reever, K., & Bach-Peterson, J. (1980). Relatives of the impaired elderly: Correlates of feelings of burden. *Gerontologist, 20*(6), 649–655

Women and Intergenerational Caregiving in Families: Structure, Ethnicity, and Building Family Ties

Carol M. Musil, Camille B. Warner, Eleanor P. Stoller, and Tanetta E. Andersson

This chapter focuses on three major aspects of caregiving between generations. In the first section, we examine women as caregivers, the historical perspectives on women and caregiving, and women's caregiving across the lifespan. Second, we consider intergenerational caregiving, especially grandmothers and the vital role they play in their families but also the interactions among generations within the family. Finally, we discuss ethnic heritage, an important dimension of family identity, and ways that families can strengthen intergenerational ties by recognizing and celebrating their cultural heritage.

WOMEN, CAREGIVING, AND FAMILIES

Families who comprise the majority of informal caregivers, are the unpaid sector of the country's health care system; they provide nearly 80% of the long-term care in the United States. This informal caregiving is usually unpaid, based on existing relationships and with little or no certified training of the caregiver. The majority of informal (as well as formal) caregivers are women; women provide most of the day-to-day, hands-on personal tasks while men are more likely to provide financial assistance or make arrangements for paid formal services, repairs, and transportation.

A report from the Senate's Special Committee on Aging (2002) meeting approximates that 75% of all caregivers are women. Informal caregivers are our mothers, aunts, sisters, nieces, wives, daughters, granddaughters and grandmothers. Women spend roughly 35 years of their lives caring for parents and children. The profile of the average caregiver is a woman aged 46 caring for a 77-year old mother. The average American woman can expect to care for one or more children for 17 years and 18 years for an elderly parent (Senate Special Committee on Aging). The average caregiver provides 18 hours a week of assistance, but there are countless caregiving arrangements.

According to a 1997 National Alliance for Caregiving (NAC) report, 23.2% of all U.S. households are involved in caregiving for elderly family members. The terms "sandwich generation" or "woman in the middle" describe 20%–40% of female caregivers providing care for an older relative and a child under the age of 18. The term "club sandwich" can be used to describe the caregiving situations of women who are assisting aging parents, minor-aged children, grandparents, and grandchildren (Senate Special Committee on Aging, 2002). The sandwich analogies are generalizations for the complex and multifaceted relationships among caregivers and the care recipients that can exist within a family.

Of the caregivers identified by the NAC report, 64.2% of caregivers were employed; 51.8% of those were employed full-time. Nearly one third of women caregivers are caring for more than one person and are married and work outside of the home. More than half of employed caregivers have had to make changes at work to accommodate their caregiving situations—such as reducing work hours, going in late, or leaving early. Naomi Gerstel (2000) uses the term the "third shift," which refers to the care work women do outside of the home (e.g., assisting neighbors, volunteering) while often doing a disproportionate share of work in the home (e.g., childcare, housework) in addition to paid work.

Historical Perspectives on Women as Caregivers

From a historical perspective, the gender system of work distribution dictates that women perform "care work" in the home, such as raising the children, providing meals for the family, and performing household tasks such as cleaning, while men should function in the work world as the family breadwinners. Interestingly, the concept of breadwinning did not emerge until the 19th century. Prior to that time, in largely agricultural societies, men and their families not only made their own bread, they grew their own grain and yeast (Williams, 2000). During that time, men were involved in the children's care; child rearing was considered too important for women to handle without help. Similarly, women helped with so-called men's work, such as gathering wood and working on the family farm.

The gender-based division of labor arose around 1780, and by the turn of the 19th century, the pattern for men to work in factories and women to work in the home had evolved (Williams, 2000). The ideology behind domesticity is that men are naturally aggressive and competitive and thus better suited for the market world, whereas women are gentler, kinder, and best suited to deal with matters of the heart, which translates into an ethic for caring and nurturing. Domesticity has changed significantly in the last several decades, as more women are in the labor force, and men have become increasingly involved in child-related care work, but the social mores and values associated with female domesticity remain in many aspects of American society. DeVault (1991, 1999) reminds us that strict domesticity has rarely been an option for the poor and for women of color because survival required that all family members (male, female, young and old) cooperate in both family and work domains.

Gerstel's (2000) review of gender and care-work presents four theoretical perspectives or causal explanations that shed light on the gender and caregiving issue: essentialist, internalization, categorical, and variation. The *essentialist* explanation suggests that caregiving and nurturing are part of the biological makeup of women. In other words, women and men are wired differently, and women naturally assume roles as caregivers within and outside their families. Women care (feel), therefore they provide care (assist); this is also known as the "ethic of care" in feminist research (Goodwin & Gibson, 2002).

Another perspective, *internalization,* assumes that boys and girls receive differential treatment and socialization in American society and thus internalize those roles and expectations that translate into behavior and personality differences. Girls are taught to care for others, while boys are taught to be tough. Gender socialization is practiced at home and reinforced in school, places of worship, and among peers and social groups, including social rituals and practices such as dating. The difference in the socialization of boys and girls becomes ingrained or internalized so that roles and expectations of the two genders are not as easily negotiated.

A third perspective, the *categorical* explanations, accept gender as a social construction based on differences in legal structure, social expectations, and power differences between men and women. In American society, men are disproportionately more powerful than women in terms of wealth and status indicators; this affords them more opportunities and choices in both the public and private arenas. Jobs help establish who should give care (Gerstel & Gallagher, 2001), which usually translates into women providing care work and men generating income. In addition, caregiving is viewed as "women's work" and is often devalued.

The last explanation, *variation,* emphasizes the influence of diversity in the structure of individual's lives. Gerstel (2000) suggests that gender influences caregiving only through other factors, especially social position (e.g., prestige, power, wealth, race/ethnicity). For instance, women in higher paid, more prestigious white-collar jobs tend to display caregiving patterns similar to those of men. Gerstel argues that the variation is the best explanation for understanding the dynamic nature of caregiving. All of these perspectives operate to varying degrees in American society, although other cultures may have additional perspectives (e.g., religious perspectives) that influence beliefs about women and caregiving.

Influences on Caregiving

Caregiving evolves over a women's life span. Women learn at a young age that care work is acceptable and frequently expected. For example, adolescent girls more often than boys begin babysitting for their own family and other families. Again in young adulthood and middle age, women bear the major responsibility for care of children, spouses, aging parents/parents-in-law, and friends, as well as for planning birthdays, holidays, and other events. As women age, they often want to—or are expected to—care for their aging spouse, adult children, grandchildren, aging friends, and relatives.

Perhaps the most profound influence on caregiving has been the changing demographics in American society. The shift in the American population's age structure has changed family relationships. The increase in the elderly population, differences in gender longevity, decreased fertility, increased numbers of women in the labor force by choice and need, and limited long-term care options has affected the when, how, and who of caregiving. As average life expectancy increases, so does the need for assistance with activities of daily living. In addition, the concept of the American family has been explicitly redefined to accommodate other relatives, nonblood or psuedo-kin, and integrated households, especially for people of color. Thus, for some American households, the empty nest has been filled by an elderly parent or parents and/or adult child or children who may be divorced or cannot maintain a home of their own. Many of these adult children bring their children or the grandchildren into the home. One type of caregiving that has been increasing over the last decade is the phenomenon of grandmothers who are caring for or raising their grandchildren because the biological parents are unable to do so due to a variety of factors, including substance abuse, incarceration, mental or physical illness, death, or military service.

Women, Caregiving, and Well-Being

Being a caregiver is a dynamic role that is often equated to a career (Pearlin, Mullan, Semple & Skaff, 1990), although some types of caregiving, such as to spouses, parents, or other relatives, is often unexpected when it occurs (although not entirely unanticipated as an eventuality in one's life) (Aneshensel, Pearlin, Mullan, Zarit, & Whitlatch, 1995). Moen, Robison, and Dempster-McClain (1995) consider the duration and timing of caregiving during the lifecycle as influencing women's well being when involved in caregiving. Others (Neugarten & Neugarten, 1987; Pearlin, McKean, & Skaff, 1996; Burton, 1996) refer to whether caregiving is an "on time" or an "off time" event, with more stress associated with "off time" than "on time" caregiving. For example, when a woman suddenly becomes a grandmother while still raising her own children, or if she must care for a spouse with early onset Alzheimer's disease, the "off-time" nature of the event may accentuate the stress of the caregiving experience. However, even relatively "on time" caregiving, such as caring for an elderly spouse with Alzheimer's disease, is difficult. There is little research in the caregiving literature that incorporates these important concepts.

When caregivers describe their experience, they often report a spectrum of emotions, ranging from burdensome and stressful to uplifting and rewarding; often, caregivers report both strain and reward simultaneously. Factors such as the circumstances of caregiving, the relationship to the care recipient, and the health and functional status of the care recipient affect the experience of caregiving for the caregiver. Caregivers of older adults often see caregiving as a responsibility, an opportunity to repay a spouse or parent, or a chance to grow closer with the care recipient. The entrance into the caregiving role can be gradual, particularly if there is no acute precipitating event such as a stroke or sudden illness. Not uncommonly, a spouse may not even be aware of taking on increasing caregiving activities; initially, he or she may think of it as compensating for the partner's deficiencies eventually recognizing his or her role as a caregiver (Perry, 2002).

Caregiving is often a drain on the caregiver's finances and physical and mental health, because caregivers often feel that they are holding down two full-time jobs. Nearly 25% of women caregivers experience health problems related to caregiving activities, and 31% of caregivers report a decrease in family savings because of caregiving responsibilities (Falik & Collins, 1996). Women are more vulnerable to poverty than men and face a higher risk of illness and disability when caregiving (Stoller, 1992).

The rewarding aspects of caregiving also must be considered when understanding women's role in care work. For many women caregivers, the caregiving experience is not only gratifying but also empowering. Gerstel (2000) found in her research on African-American and Euro-American women that African-American women engaged in caregiving for empowerment as well as survival. These women of color found a role where they not only fulfilled an essential function but also felt valued and appreciated despite their otherwise less powerful membership in American society. Caring can be an empowering activity that results from helping others and making them happy (Bubeck, 2002).

Families, and Caregiving to Grandparents

An area with great significance that has received little attention is the family's response to the caregiving. The caregiving situation can be especially challenging to the family because it requires that the caregiver divert some time from her or his own family. Frequently, difficult decisions about living arrangements must be addressed with the grandparent/care recipient's immediate and extended family.

If the grandparent is living at the home of an adult child, the caregiving situation may require uncomfortable changes in living arrangements and alterations in the family's usual patterns of functioning and interacting. In addition, grandchildren, when watching a health decline in a grandparent, may be confronted with complex and unfamiliar feelings they had not previously experienced. Children, who take many behavioral cues from parents, are often quite responsive to dealing with these challenges, especially when supported in doing so.

Finding ways to help grandchildren maintain relatedness when grandparents are ill or impaired is important for both the younger and older generations, even if it requires carving out time for the generations to be together. Supporting kids in understanding the health changes in the older adults who are close to them provides important lessons about themselves and about caregivers and their families. Placing health changes within the context of normality, integrating the changes in the family's ways of functioning, and maintaining a sense of continuity and order are often suggested as ways to maintain family functioning during stressful circumstances, such as caregiving. Limited research about the effectiveness and application of these approaches in caregiving families has been reported to date, so the literature provides inadequate guidance on these practical issues.

GRANDMOTHERS, FAMILIES AND CAREGIVING

The role of grandparents is being reemphasized in the United States (Cox, 2000). In many families, grandparents occupy background, supportive roles, providing love, money, and occasional caregiving help within families, but during times of hardship, grandparents may function as a safety valve and take on a more central role if needed (Cherlin & Furstenberg, 1986). Grandparents can provide a continuum of care that ranges from those grandparents who have (1) primary/custodial responsibility for one or more grandchildren, (2) grandparents who, in conjunction with children's parents, provide care for grandchildren in a multigenerational household, (3) grandparents who provide extensive daycare or babysitting for grandchildren, and (4) those grandparents with no day-to-day caregiving to grandchildren but who have an active interest in their grandchildren's lives, regardless of their proximity to grandchildren.

Issues Facing Grandparents Raising Their Grandchildren

Over the past three decades, there has been a dramatic increase in grandparents assuming caregiving roles. According to the U.S. Census Bureau, from 1970 to 1997, the number of American children living in a household maintained by a grandparent rose by 76% (Lugalia, 1998). Thus, in 1997, some 3.7 million grandparents were raising their grandchildren. Increases in substance abuse, incarceration, teen pregnancy, and AIDS coupled with under funding for mental health care have affected families and children, which in turn has led to grandparents assuming a greater caregiving role. Such caregiving is consistent with a public policy emphasis on family preservation.

Of the 3.7 million grandparents raising their grandchildren, 2.3 million are grandmother-headed households. Of the children being raised by grandparents, 13.5% are African American, 6.5% are Hispanics and 4.1% are White non-Hispanic (Casper & Bryson, 1998). Among all family types, grandmothers maintaining households alone are much more likely than grandparents in other family types to face economic hardship. For example, in 2000, the mean household income of grandmother-only households with no parents present was only $19,750, compared with $61,632 for households with both grandparents and one or both parents of the grandchildren present. Grandmothers maintaining households alone, with no spouse or parents present, are also much less likely than other grandparent householders to be in the labor force (Casper & Bryson, 1998).

For grandmothers raising grandchildren who are employed outside the home, many must find day care for grandchildren, which adds to financial stress, while others reduce work hours or quit working to manage the family situation. Not all grandmothers raising grandchildren receive financial support for grandchildren. If there is no formal custody arrangement, it may be difficult for children to receive health and educational services for grandchildren. A number of states have initiatives for helping grandparents raising grandchildren receive services and support, such as the Navigator Program in the state of Ohio, but these programs are vulnerable to budget cuts.

Grandmothers raising grandchildren face all the challenges encountered by parents, as well as some additional ones. Caring for grandchildren full time may be especially difficult as the grandmothers are frequently developing their own health problems, and many report fatigue in trying to keep up with the grandchildren's activities. In the words of one grandmother:

> Tried to practice what I have learned from Stephen Covey's *The 7 Habits of Highly Effective People* . . . The change in routine, the wait at the doctor's office, the kids not being able to find their shin guards, the two oldest siblings fighting, and my cold create the most unpleasant of days. Even Stephen Covey would have cracked under the pressure.

Grandmothers raising grandchildren report more parenting stress than mothers, and also more personal distress (Musil, Young-blut, Ahn, & Curry, 2002). The older the grandchildren, the greater the stress. While younger children may be more physically demanding, older children present more difficult social, behavioral, and academic issues. Further, respite and other programs may be available for grandmothers raising younger grandchildren, but there may be fewer such options for those raising older grandchildren. Issues related to drug and alcohol use present concerns for grandparents raising grandchildren. If the children have been exposed to drugs or alcohol prenatally, they may have attention disorders, behavior problems, or health problems that require special services.

Grandparents who are primary caregivers for their grandchildren often encounter a number of school-related issues. Approximately one third of grandchildren may need to change schools when they move in with a grandparent, so these children may experience additional stress related to not having friends nearby when they relocate. Helping grandchildren with homework can also be a real challenge.

Multigenerational Homes

Recent data on multigenerational homes indicate a similar rise. Data from the 2000 census indicate that there are some 2.6 million multigenerational households with a combination of grandparents, parent, grandchild and even great grandparents in the United States (U.S. Census Bureau, 2001). The reasons for this increase in multigenerational homes can be traced to a number of circumstances, such as substance use and abuse, teenage pregnancy, financial instability, marital disruptions, and divorce. Mutual agreements between generations sometimes lead to a multigenerational living arrangement. For example, grandparents and parents may enter a partnership, mapping out roles and functions to be performed by specific members in the household. In such an arrangement, grandmothers may take care of the children while the parents work; in other cases, the adult children may move back to the grandparents' home after divorce or if one of the parents is separated by distance due to work or military obligations. Multigenerational households also may reflect important cultural variations. Multigenerational homes tend to be more common among families of color, and families of recent immigrants (Simmons & Dye, 2003).

Other Grandmothers

Grandparents who live apart from grandchildren, the most common arrangement in the United States, experience the rewards of having grandchildren, without the day-to-day hassles. If grandparents live close enough to grandchildren, they may take the children to appointments, attend children's school activities and extracurricular events, or provide occasional babysitting for them. Not infrequently, grandparents take on the role of primary day-care provider/babysitter for the grandchildren while the adult children work or attend school. Some of these grandparents may have ambivalence about their responsibilities and restrictions on their time but feel pressure to continue their daily involvement. For many women, grandmotherhood is only one dimension of their identity.

BUILDING INTERGENERATIONAL TIES

Ethnic heritage provides a perspective that can strengthen intergenerational relationships within families, including the provision of care for frail elderly relatives. Often, when gerontologists speak about ethnicity, we limit our attention to so-called minority groups or perhaps recent immigrants to the United States. But ethnicity can be a resource for a broader spectrum of families, including the descendants of immigrants from different parts of Europe.

A distinction is sometimes made between ethnicity from *outside* and ethnicity from *inside*. Viewed from outside, ethnicity is an attribution on the basis of which a viewer makes certain assumptions about another person. For example, people often think they can identify a person's ethnic heritage on the basis of a physical feature, surname, or residential history. Viewed from inside, ethnicity is a basis for group identification and belonging, a way of life, and a shared identity that provides a sense of distinctiveness from other groups. Noel Chrisman (1970), studying Danish-Americans in California, argued that fellow ethnics are in some ways "known in advance." As one third-generation Finnish-American (Stoller, 1996) explained, "You can meet a complete stranger and find out that they're Finnish and all of a sudden there's an instant bond. . . . For some reason, if they're a Finn, that makes them OK." In their studies of second- and third-generation European Americans, the sociologists Richard Alba (1990) and Mary Waters (1990) found a sense of affinity among people of similar ethnic background, which they described as a feeling of communality or even kinship.

Ethnicity implies a shared history and a common place of geographical origin. It can lead to special interests about politics in the homeland and in the United States. Common ethnicity implies a similar culture that includes the same language or dialect, shared folklore, music, food preferences, and holiday observances. Often, there are other organizational ties, such as membership in lodges, associations and groups, and similar religious preferences. Sometimes fellow ethnics share a common residence within an ethnic community. Even among elders who no longer live in ethnic neighborhoods, ethnic neighborhoods of their childhood are fondly remembered as environments that provided warmth and support (Waters, 1990).

Knowledge of ethnic history and heritage can buffer the loss of status that occurs in late life (Luborsky & Rubenstein, 1987). A revival of interest in ethnicity, particularly among younger generations, can increase the self-esteem of the older generation and provide them with an exchange resource. To the extent that the aged are viewed as repositories of knowledge or expertise on ethnicity and to the extent that this knowledge is prized by other people, then the status of older people is enhanced because they are perceived as sources of valuable information (Weibel-Orlando, 1988). Tracing ethnic traditions within families also provides a context for life review, as older people look back on childhood memories of immigrant parents or grandparents.

Too often, younger family members are unaware of the benefits of learning about ethnic heritage and either tune out or become irritated with older relatives who repeat stories from the past.

Practitioners can strengthen family ties by helping younger relatives understand that reminiscing by older people is not just living in
the past—it is a way to provide coherence and meaning to one's life.

These advantages of ethnicity are strongest when a person lives in
close proximity to coethnics (i.e., others with the same ethnic background). Living within an area of ethnic residential concentration
increases the likelihood that social contacts will place older people
in contact with fellow ethnics. Residential concentration can support an ethnic infrastructure and intensify ethnic cultural experiences, a phenomenon Alba (1990) describes as the "supply side of
ethnicity." By highlighting the visibility of an ethnic group, supply
side features of ethnic communities enhance the attraction of an
ethnic identity and foster a sense of loyalty and attachment to the
group (Litwak & Silverstein, 1991).

But ethnicity can sometimes be a barrier for older people who are
isolated from fellow ethnics. Service providers are frequently unaware
of important cultural traditions. Ethnic newspapers, churches and
temples, and radio programs are rare. Finding appropriate foods
can be difficult. Language often becomes a barrier. Even people
who develop fluency in English can lose some of this fluency after
a stroke. This is more a problem in the United States than in some
other societies, because Americans expect people to be fluent in
English.

So how can we apply this understanding of ethnicity in late life to
strengthening the bonds within our families? One of the most
important areas in which ethnicity can be applied is in the process
of life review. Grandparents and other elderly relatives may be wor-
ried about the stereotypes of living in the past and seem reluctant to
begin reviewing their lives. Some may even be hesitant to share certain aspects of their lives because of the fear of being shamed
and/or judged by other family members. Younger family members
should encourage life review projects with the elders of the family.
These collected reminiscences provide a meaningful legacy for
their survivors.

Memories can be sparked in a number of ways. Sorting boxes of
old photographs or souvenirs often jogs memories, as does listening
to an old record, looking at old newspaper clippings or magazines,
or reading short stories about the past. Historical events also trigger
memories. Watching a video set in a particular place and particular
time can generate discussions if families encourage their elderly relative to "tell us what it was like to live back then?" The senses are

powerful catalysts as well. The smell of baking bread, the feel of crayons or a baseball, the sound of a foghorn can trigger a flood of memories.

When using reminiscence as a mechanism for life review, historical accuracy is not so important, as events that occurred 50, 60, or more years ago are recalled. In the case of second-generation informants, reports may be second-hand. People forget many details of everyday life. Over the years, they may have partially rewritten their biographies, rationalizing or revising the past to conform to their self-concepts. But this is an important part of the life review process. It is important to explore the feelings or subjective impact of these experiences. When an elderly woman tells us today how she felt 60 years ago when someone made fun of her "unpronounceable" last name, we learn something about the long-term significance of this experience even if she may have exaggerated its frequency.

A second implication of the research on aging and ethnicity is the importance of sharing ethnic heritage, which, as indicated above, reinforces continuity with the past. If the older person assumes the role of teacher, it enhances the older person's self-esteem and strengthens intergenerational relationships. Sharing can be encouraged through a variety of strategies; for example, by engaging in the following activities: (1) creating a cookbook of ethnic recipes, including special holiday dishes, (2) teaching young people how to make seasonal decorations or to do "handwork" like sewing or knitting, (3) Translating words of folk songs—or contemporary rock music—from the country of origin, (4) finding out about famous people, either historical figures or contemporary ones (professional athletes, politicians, actors), from the same ethnic background, (5) learning a few words of the language of origin, which can be part of a "secret" language within the family, and (6) starting a family tree and tracking down possible relatives or locating new pen pals in the area where immigrant ancestors were born. A number of sources of information are available to assist families in drawing on their ethnic heritage as a caregiving resource. Bookstores and libraries stock a variety of guides to writing family narratives. Many communities have chapters of national ethnic organizations. Searching the Internet for hyphenated ethnic labels (e.g., Italian-American, Swedish-American) provides links to a variety of ethnically based organizations and informational resources. Motivating children and teens to participate in such projects can be enhanced when families can link ethnic activities to children's current interests ("Did you know that hockey player is from Norway—not too far from where your great grandmother was born? Do you think he knows any of our relatives?"), or school assignments ("Your grandma was a little girl during the Great Depression. Maybe you could interview her for part of your history paper.") But even without enthusiastic children or grandchildren, reflecting on the family's ethnic heritage can provide a context for listening to elderly relatives as they narrate their identities and, in the process, create a family legacy for generations who might otherwise forget their historic origins.

SUMMARY

Women's roles in caregiving across the generations take many forms. Throughout the course of their lives, women have cared for many people. They have also functioned as leaders in their churches and communities and role models in professional careers. This care work is not new to women, but the extent of responsibility that women now assume for the care of elders has dramatically increased during this past century as people are living longer and with more disabilities, frequently concomitant with working outside the home. Changes in family composition have contributed to more young, middle aged, and older women engaging in caregiving—often at unexpected periods in their lives. Throughout this process, women are often responsible for passing on family traditions and weaving ethnic and cultural heritage into the family life story.

Women have balanced the many responsibilities in their lives to provide these many types of care and assistance to family members and friends. Mutual support and understanding between the younger and older generations about the unique contributions of each family member fosters respect and strengthens the family bond.

REFERENCES

Alba, R. (1990). *Ethnic identity: The transformation of white America.* New Haven: Yale University Press.
Aneshensel, C., Pearlin, L., Mullan, J., Zarit, S., & Whitlatch, C. (1995). *Profiles in caregiving: The unexpected career.* San Diego: Academic Press.
Angier, N. (1997, September 16). Theorists see evolutionary advantages in menopause. *The New York Times,* Section F, p. 1, col. 4.

Bubeck, D. G. (2002). Justice and the labor of care. In E. Kittay & E. Feder (Eds.), *The subject of care: Feminist perspectives on dependency.* Lanham, MD: Rowman & Littlefield Publishers.

Burton, L. M. (1996). Age norms, the timing of family role transitions, and intergenerational caregiving among aging African American women. *Gerontologist, 36*(2), 199–208.

Casper, L. M., & Bryson, K. R. (1998, March). *Co-resident grandparents and their grandchildren: Grandparent-maintained families.* U.S. Bureau of the Census, Population Division Working Paper No. 26.

Cherlin, A., & Furstenberg, F. (1986). *New American grandparent: A place in the family, a life apart.* New York: Basic Books.

Chrisman, N. J. (1970). Situation and social network in cities. *The Canadian Review of Sociology and Anthropology, 7*(4), 245–257.

Cox, C. (Ed.). (2000). *To grandmother's house we go and stay: Perspectives on custodial grandparents.* New York: Springer Publishing.

De Vault, M. (1991). *Feeding the family: The social organization of caring as gendered work.* Chicago: University of Chicago Press.

DeVault, M. (1999). *Liberating method: Feminism and social research.* Philadelphia: Temple University Press.

Falik, M., & Collins, K. (1996). *Women's health: The Commonwealth Fund Survey.* Baltimore: Johns Hopkins University Press.

Gerstel, N. (2000). The third shift: Gender and care work outside the home. *Qualitative Sociology, 23*(4), 467–483

Gerstel, N., & Gallagher, S. (2001). Men's caregiving, gender, and the contingent character of care. *Gender & Society, 15*(2), 197–217.

Goodwin, R., & Gibson, D. (2002) The decasualization of eldercare. In E. Kittay & E. Feder (Eds.), *The subject of care: Feminist perspectives on dependency.* Lanham, MD: Rowman & Littlefield Publishers..

Litwak, E., & Silverstein, M. (1991). Helping networks among the Jewish elderly. *Contemporary Jewry, 11*(3), 3–50.

Luborsky, M., & Rubenstein, R., (1987). Ethnicity and lifetimes: Self-concepts and situational contexts of ethnic identity in late life. In D. Gelfand & D. Barressi (Eds.), *Ethnic dimensions of aging* (pp. 35–50). New York: Springer Publishing.

Lugaila, T. (1998). *Marital Status and Living Arrangements: March 1997.* Bureau of the Census, Current Population Reports (forthcoming).

Moen, P., Robison, J., & Dempster-Mclain, D. (1995). Caregiving and women's well-being: A life course approach. *Journal of Health and Social Behavior, 36*(3), 259–273.

Musil, C., Youngblut, J., Ahn, S., & Curry, V. (2002). Parenting stress: A comparison of grandmother caretakers and mothers. *Journal of Mental Health and Aging, 8*(3), 197–210.

National Alliance for Caregiving (NAC). (1998). *The caregiving boom: Baby boomer women giving care.* Bethesda, MD. Retrieved from http://www.caregiving.org/babyboomer.pdf

Neugarten, B., & Neugarten, D. (1987). Changing meanings of age. *Psychology Today, 21*(5), 29–30.

Pearlin, L., Mullan, J., Semple, S., & Skaff, M. (1990). Caregiving and the stress process: An overview of concepts and their measures. *The Gerontologist, 30*(5), 583–591.

Pearlin, L. I., & McKean Skaff, M. (1996). Stress and the life course: A paradigmatic alliance. *The Gerontologist, 36*(2), 239–247.

Perry, J. (2002). Wives giving care to husbands with Alzheimer's disease: A process of interpretive caring. *Research in Nursing and Health, 25*(4), 307–316.

Roszak, T. (1998). *America the wise: The longevity revolution and the true wealth of nations.* New York: Houghton Mifflin.

Senate Special Committee on Aging. (2002, February 6). *Women and aging: Bearing the burden of long-term care.* S. Hrg. 107–291. Retrieved from http://www.access.gpo.gov/congress/senate/senate22.html

Simmons, T., & Dye, J. (2003). *Grandparents living with grandchildren: 2000 Census 2000 brief.* C2KBR-31.

Stoller, E. (1992) Gender differences in the experiences of caregiving spouses. In J. Dwyer & R. Coward (Eds.), *Gender, families and elder care* (pp. 49–64). Thousand Oaks, CA: Sage.

Stoller, E. (1996). Sauna, sisu, sibelius: Ethnic identity among Finnish Americans. *Sociological Quarterly, 37*(1), 145–175.

U.S. Census Bureau. (2001). *Multigenerational Households for the United States, States, and Puerto Rico: 2000.* Retrieved from http://www.census.gov/population/cen2000/phc-t17.pdf

Waters, M. (1990). *Ethnic options: Choosing identities in America.* Berkeley: University of California Press.

Weibel-Orlando, J. (1988). Indians, ethnicity as a resource, and aging: You can go home again. *Journal of Cross-Cultural Gerontology, 3*(4), 323–348.

Williams, J. (2000). *Unbending gender: Why family and work conflict and what to do about it.* Oxford, England: Oxford University Press.

CHAPTER 9

Effects of a Montessori-Based Intergenerational Program on Engagement and Affect for Adult Day Care Clients With Dementia

Cameron J. Camp, Silvia Orsulic-Jeras, Michelle M. Lee, and Katherine S. Judge

Within the past two decades, an increased focus has been placed on the provision of meaningful activities for persons with Alzheimer's disease (AD) and related dementias (Alzheimer's Association, 1995; Beck, Zgola, & Shue, 2000; Bowlby, 1993; Buettner, 1999; Buettner et al., 1996; Camp, 1999; Dawson, Wells, & Kline, 1993; Dreher, 1997; Fazio, Chavin, & Clair, 1999; Hellen, 1998; Judge, Camp, & Orsulic-Jeras, 2000; Laurenhue, 2000; Orsulic-Jeras, Judge, & Camp, 2000; Orsulic-Jeras, Schneider, & Camp, 2000; Orsulic-Jeras, Schneider, Camp, Nicholson, & Helbig, 2001; Plautz & Camp, 2000; Volicer & Bloom-Charette, 1999; Zgola, 1987). One such form of meaningful activity is intergenerational programming between older adults with dementia and young children. In appropriately structured programming, older adults with dementia are given an opportunity to utilize their social skills by acting as mentors, and young children are provided with a chance to demonstrate prosocial behaviors towards the elderly while learning new skills (Camp et al., 1997; Dellmann-Jenkins, Lamber, & Fruit, 1991). Intergenerational programming has been found to increase levels of social interaction and decrease solitary behaviors among adult day-care members (Short-Degraff & Diamond, 1996). Similarly,

159

long-term care residents with dementia working with young children have shown an increase in spontaneous positive behaviors, and, in turn, a decrease in subsequent levels of agitation (Newman & Ward, 1992–1993; Ward, Los Kamp, & Newman, 1996).

Although the advantages of intergenerational programming for persons with dementia are clear, implementing effective intergenerational activities can be challenging. First, requirements of a successful intergenerational program specify that the activities be meaningful for both groups of participants (Griff et al., 1996; Dellmann-Jenkins, 1997). Second, once meaningful activities are selected, it is imperative that they demonstrate the ability to engage both older adults and young children over a sustained period of time. Identifying such tasks can be difficult for staff members who may have limited experience in working with both age groups concurrently (Griff et al., 1996). Finally, intergenerational activities that are successful for one group of older adults (community-dwelling elderly) are not necessarily appropriate for other groups (frail elderly, elderly with Alzheimer's disease), and can result in negative responses from older adults, children, and staff (Griff et al., 1996).

Selecting appropriate activities is a cardinal component of adult day-care programs for persons with dementia. Difficult or nonengaging activities can lead to an increase in behavioral problems, while appropriate and appealing activities can lead to a decrease in behavior problems in persons with dementia (Acello, 1997; Aronstein, Olson, & Schulman, 1996, Buettner, 1999; Vance, Camp, & Kabacof, 1996). In recent years, researchers and staff who work with cognitively impaired older adults have attempted to create activities that would be especially suitable to the specific needs of this population (Judge, Camp, & Orsulic-Jeras, 2000; Orsulic-Jeras, Judge, & Camp, 2000; Orsulic-Jeras, Schneider, & Camp, 2000; Orsulic-Jeras, Schneider, Camp, Nicholson, & Helbig, 2001; Stevens, Camp, King, Bailey, & Hsu, 1998; Stevens, King, & Camp, 1993). In particular, these researchers have emphasized the use of Montessori-based activities for persons with dementia.

MONTESSORI-BASED ACTIVITIES
FOR PERSONS WITH DEMENTIA

The Montessori method of education for children, developed by Maria Montessori, emphasizes (1) structured use of everyday materials, (2) breakdown of tasks into simpler steps, (3) subsequent progression of simpler tasks to more complex ones, if and when appropriate, and (4) developmental sequencing of tasks (Judge, Camp, & Orsulic-Jeras, 2000; Orsulic-Jeras, Judge, & Camp, 2000; Orsulic-Jeras, Schneider, & Camp, 2000; Orsulic-Jeras, Schneider, Camp, Nicholson, & Helbig, 2001). Montessori-based activities are believed to be especially useful for individuals with dementia, since activities involve familiar objects, are self-correcting, utilize procedural/nondeclarative rather than declarative memory (Squire, 1992, 1994), and can be easily modified to adjust to the individual's level of functioning (Camp, 1999). Further, materials used in the creation of Montessori-based activities provide cognitive and sensory stimulation, practice with skills necessary to maintain independence, and encourage the expression of remaining verbal and social skills (Camp, 1999; Orsulic-Jeras et al., 2001).

Past research has shown that while participating in Montessori-based individual and small group activities, persons with dementia have demonstrated a significant increase in levels of constructive engagement and a decrease in their levels of passive engagement and sleeping in comparison to their performance in regularly scheduled activities programming (Judge, Camp, & Orsulic-Jeras, 2000; Orsulic-Jeras, Judge, & Camp, 2000; Orsulic-Jeras, Schneider, & Camp, 2000). In addition, a previous pilot study conducted using Montessori-based methods with residents of a special care unit demonstrated that older adults with dementia could successfully teach Montessori-based activities to young children, with the levels of disengagement shown by these older adults decreasing as a result of the program (Camp et al., 1997).

The Benefits of Montessori-Based Activities in Intergenerational Programming

Given the success of Montessori activities for young children and older adults with dementia, their implementation into intergenerational programming within adult day care settings shows considerable promise (Camp et al., 1997). Montessori-based activities generally involve acquiring knowledge and skills associated with everyday living. Older adults with cognitive impairments can tap into their existing lifelong experience to help children master such tasks. Also, older adults can give guidance and praise to children, providing a meaningful social role as a mentor or teacher. Children, as well, can enjoy gaining new knowledge and demonstrating mastery of new skills acquired from their older adult "teachers."

Thus, Montessori-based activities appear to provide a promising avenue for intergenerational programming between adult day care members and young children. The purpose of the present study was to demonstrate the effectiveness of Montessori-based activities in intergenerational programming between adult day care members and preschool age children. Specifically, it was hypothesized that adult day care members would be more constructively engaged and would demonstrate less disengagement from scheduled activities when participating in Montessori-based intergenerational programming (treatment condition), compared to regularly scheduled adult day care activities (control condition). In addition, it was also hypothesized that participants in the treatment condition would exhibit more positive affect and less negative affect when compared to the control condition.

METHOD

Participants

The study was conducted at Menorah Park Center for Senior Living, an extended-care facility providing independent living, assisted living, long-term care, and adult day-care services in Beachwood, Ohio, a suburb of Cleveland. Thirteen children from Menorah Park's FUNdamentals child-care center, ranging in age from 2.5 to 5 years old, participated in the study.

Twenty clients from its adult day-care center were initially recruited. In order to participate in the study, participants had to have a diagnosis of dementia, be English speaking, and attend adult day care on a regular basis. Exclusion criteria included a Mini-Mental State Exam (MMSE) (Folstein et al., 1975) score of less than 10. Five participants were dropped from the study for not meeting inclusion criteria ($n = 4$) or because they were no longer attending the day center ($n = 1$). Thus, 15 older adult participants (11 women and 4 men) completed the study. Their MMSE scores ranged from 10 to 25 ($M = 17$, $SD = 4.86$). Age ranged from 50 to 95 years ($M = 80.57$, $SD = 11.93$). Eighty-seven percent of the participants were Caucasian and 13% were African-American. Seventy-seven percent of participants had an education level of high school or less, and 23% had completed at least some college coursework. Regarding diagnosis of dementia, 33.3% had probable Alzheimer's disease (AD), 13.3% had probable vascular dementia, and 53.3% had mixed or other types of dementia.

Older participants were randomly assigned to two groups. Group 1 would initially take part in Montessori-based intergenerational programming. Group 2 would receive such programming in the second half of the study. Analyses were conducted to examine group differences on the variables of age, gender, ethnicity, level of education, type of dementia diagnosis, and MMSE score. Independent t-tests revealed no significant differences in age or MMSE scores between these two groups ($t < 1$). Chi-square analyses showed no significant group differences in level of education or type of dementia diagnosis.

Screening

All older adult and child participants were administered the Myers Menorah Park/Montessori Assessment System (MMP/MAS), a qualitative Montessori-based assessment system that includes seven specific Montessori activities designed to assess an individual's remaining cognitive, motor, sensory, and social abilities (Camp, Koss, & Judge, 1999; Orsulic-Jeras, Judge & Camp, 2000). The MMP/MAS was given to assess the participants' levels of these abilities and to determine what types of Montessori programming would be most likely to appeal them.

Materials and Procedures

Participants were assigned to groups by finding pairs of adult day-care clients who were similar in their MMSE scores; then, one member of each pair was randomly assigned to either Group 1 or Group 2. Group 1 ($n = 8$) was assigned to participate in the treatment condition (Montessori-based intergenerational programming) first, whereas Group 2 ($n = 7$) was initially observed in the control condition (regularly scheduled adult day center activities). Utilizing a crossover design, the groups switched midway through the study, with Group 1 receiving the control condition and Group 2 participating in Montessori-based intergenerational programming in the second half (phase) of the study. Each treatment and control condition phase lasted 6 months for each group, such that the entire study lasted one year.

Observational Data/Outcome Measures

Observational data were gathered using the Myers Research Institute Engagement Scale (MRI-ES; Judge, Camp, & Orsulic-Jeras, 2000;

Orsulic-Jeras, Judge, & Camp, 2000), and the Affect Rating Scale (ARS; Lawton, Van Haitsma, & Klapper, 1996; Lawton, Van Haitsma, Perkinson, & Ruckdeschel, 1999). Both of these measures are described next.

Engagement. The MRI-ES measures the amount and type of engagement exhibited by individuals participating in activities. Four main categories of engagement are measured through direct observation: constructive engagement (CE), active engagement (AE), passive engagement (PE), and nonengagement (NE).

CE is defined as any motor or verbal behavior exhibited in response to the activity in which the client is taking part. Examples of CE could include talking in a discussion group, singing or dancing to music, or imitating the movements of the group leader during an exercise program. PE is defined as listening and/or looking behavior exhibited in response to the activity in which the client is participating. Listening to a discussion or a speaker, watching others doing exercises, watching television, and listening to music could all be coded as PE.

AE is similar to CE, except that it is not focused on the activity at hand. An example of AE would be talking to another day-center client during an exercise activity, rather than paying attention to the activity leader's directions. The fourth and final type of engagement, NE, is defined as staring off into space or another direction away from the activity, sleeping, or similar behaviors indicating lack of attention to the target activity.

Raters recorded participants' engagement during 5-minute observation windows using a handheld event recorder, the Psion Organiser II (Psion, London, U.K.), which was used with the Observer software package (Noldus Information Technology, 1995). This equipment is used to create a sequenced record of behavior codes and the length of time in seconds spent in each code. Two days a week, observations were taken of participants at three different times of day—before intergenerational programming began in the adult day center, *during* the time when some of the participants were taking part in intergenerational programming (while the other control participants were taking part in regular adult day-center activities), and *after* intergenerational programming had been completed within the center. In our analyses, this is referred to as our "Time of Programming" factor.

Affect Ratings. Affect data were recorded immediately after the 5-minute window. For the purposes of the present study, we utilized 4 affect states from the ARS (Lawton, Van Haitsma, & Klapper, 1996; Lawton, Van Haitsma, Perkinson, & Ruckdeschel, 1999): Pleasure, Anxiety/Fear, and Sadness. The time intervals that each affect could occur were: Never (1), <16 seconds (2), 16–59 seconds (3), or 1–5 minutes (4).

Treatment and Control Conditions

Regular Adult Day Care Programming. Regularly scheduled adult day-care activity programming served as the control condition against which the effects of intergenerational programming were compared. Programming at the adult day-care center consisted of a variety of individual and small and large group activities led by activities staff or volunteers. Some of these activities included music and art therapies, other musical programs, exercise, watching movies, playing cards, and discussion groups. Special activities, such as religious or holiday programming, were scheduled as well. Often, there was more than one activity going on at the same time, and clients had a choice of which activity to attend. Given the high quality and frequency of activities programming provided by the center, we did not expect to see large amounts of NE or SE in our participants. Our primary expectation was that we might see more CE and less PE during Montessori-based intergenerational programming than at other times, since such intergenerational programming usually requires that participants be actively manipulating materials and verbalizing with children during such programming.

Montessori-Based Intergenerational Programming. Montessori-based intergenerational programming served as our "treatment." This intergenerational programming was scheduled to fit within the preexisting activity times of the day center. Two to three older adult-child dyads worked simultaneously with research staff on a variety of Montessori-based tasks of the dyads' choice. A Montessori activities cabinet was created and filled with different activities designed to engage both child and older adult. Programming sessions lasted about 20 minutes, during which dyads typically worked together on three different Montessori activities. During each session, the researcher helped facilitate dyad interactions. However, the goal was to have the older adult and the child work together with as little input from the researcher as possible. Typically, the older adults' interactions with the children involved an adult assisting a child in completing Montessori activities while also informally socializing with the child. Comparisons made between observations taken during regular adult day-care programming and Montessori-based intergenerational programming are referred to as our "Type of Programming" factor.

Study Design

Data were analyzed using a 2 x 2 x 3 mixed model ANOVA design. This involved the between-subjects factor "group" (received Montessori-based intergenerational programming first and regular adult day-care programming second within the crossover design versus received Montessori-based intergenerational programming second and regular adult day-care programming first within the crossover design) and two within-subject factors: "Type of Programming" (regular adult day-care programming versus Montessori-based intergenerational programming) and "Time of Observation" (before, during, and after the intergenerational programming time period).

RESULTS

For each participant within each group and within each type of programming, a mean score was computed for all observations taken in the time periods before, during, and after introduction of intergenerational programming within the adult day-care center. Thus, each participant had six scores for each engagement and affect measure: a before, during, and after score for those occasions when the participant served in a control group condition, and a before, during, and after score for those occasions when the same participant served in the intergenerational programming condition. The group effect, in essence, was used to determine whether the order in which participants took part in control or treatment conditions influenced outcomes. Results will be discussed in terms of effects on engagement measures and effects on affect measures. Given the number of analyses conducted, no outcomes with significance levels above $p < .01$ are reported as significant.

Effects on Engagement

Our first major hypothesis was that involvement in Montessori-based intergenerational programming would produce more constructive engagement and less disengagement in planned center activities than involvement in regular adult day-care programming for participants with dementia. This hypothesis, in general, was confirmed.

CE. A significant main effect for of type of programming, F (1,13) = 93.0, $p < .001$ was found for CE. In addition, a significant main effect for time of observation, F (2,26) = 76.9, $p < .001$, was found for CE. However, these main effects were mitigated due to the presence of a significant interaction between these two factors for CE, F (2,26) = 90.2, $p < .001$. Means associated with these effects are shown in Table 9.1.

These means were compared using paired t-tests examining differences between participants' observed CE intervals when taking part in Montessori-based intergenerational programming or standard day-care programming at each time of observation. Examining the means in Table 9.1, there was little CE observed in the time period before children were introduced into the center. This was a "start-up" time period, when cars and buses bringing clients would arrive, clients would congregate in a common room, and announcements of the day's activities were given.

With regard to type of programming, similar amounts of CE were observed in the *before* time period. Similarly, no significant type of programming differences were found in amounts of CE observed in the *after* time period. However, a significant type of programming effect was seen in the time period, $t(14) = 13.1$, $p < .001$. Participants showed substantially more CE when working with children than when engaged in standard day care activities at this time period.

Passive Engagement (PE). There was a significant main effect for type of programming for PE, F (1,13) = 30.2, $p < .001$. However, a significant effect also was found for the interaction Type of Programming x Time of Observation, F (2,26) = 11.5, $p < .001$. Means associated with these effects are shown in Table 9.1. As was the case with CE, these means were compared using paired *t*-tests examining differences between participants' observed PE intervals when taking part in Montessori-based intergenerational programming or standard day-care programming at each time of observation.

TABLE 9.1   Means (and *SDs*) Seconds of Observed Engagement Scores as a Function of Type of Programming and Time of Observation

Type of Engagement	Time of Observation	Type of Programming	
		Montessori-Based Intergenerational	Regular Programming
CE	Before	0.48 (1.3)	0.29 (0.9)
	During	213.0 (35.3)	60.1 (49.3)
	After	69.9 (53.6)	74.0 (53.2)
PE	Before	137.3 (63)	148.5 (64)
	During	77.4 (32)	155.3 (67)
	After	134.2 (53)	148.7 (45)
AE	Before	86.7 (35)	87.9 (38)
	During	1.4 (1)	14.7 (13)
	After	19.9 (18)	29.3 (38)
NE	Before	32.0 (13)	21.5 (37)
	During	2.8 (9)	39.2 (53)
	After	50.7 (70)	35.2 (57)

Examining the means in Table 9.1, in most circumstances PE was observed for roughly half of the observation period, regardless of when observations were taken. When participants were in the before and after time periods, their levels of PE were not significantly different regardless of whether they received regular group programming or intergenerational programming that day. However, a significant type of programming effect was seen in the *during* time period, $t(14)$ 4.8, $p < .001$. Participants showed substantially less PE when working with children than when engaged in standard day care activities at this time period.

Finally, a significant main effect for group (received Montessori-based intergenerational programming in the first half of the program or in the second half of the program) was found for PE, $F(1,13) = 8.9$ $p < .01$. Participants who received intergenerational programming in the first part of the study showed slightly higher overall PE ($M = 155.6$ sec; $SD = 22.6$) than participants who received intergenerational programming in the second part of the study ($M = 108.3$ sec; $SD = 38.0$). However, there were no significant interactions between group and any other factor for PE, nor was the group effect nor any interaction with group significant for any other engagement measures.

Active Engagement (AE). As shown in Table 9.1, AE was a relatively low frequency event. The main effect of type of programming only approached significance by our criterion, F (1,13) = 5.7, p < .03. A significant main effect for time of observation was found, F (2,26) = 39.5, p < .001. In both types of programming, AE was highest in the early morning, lowest in the middle morning, and rose again in the latest time of observation.

Paired *t*-tests showed no significant differences for type of programming in the before and after time periods. However, a significant type of programming effect was seen in the during time period, t(14) 3.8, p < .002. Participants showed substantially less AE when working with children than when engaged in standard day-care activities at this time period. In fact, AE was rarely seen at all during intergenerational programming.

NE. There was a significant interaction between Type of Programming x Time of Observation for NE, F (2,26) = 8.8, p < .001. Means associated with these effects are shown in Table 9.1. Again, these means were first compared using paired *t*-tests examining differences between participants' observed PE intervals when taking part in Montessori-based intergenerational programming or standard day-care programming at each time of observation. Examining the means in Table 9.1, in most circumstances NE was a low frequency event, regardless of when observations were taken.

When participants were in the before and after time periods, their levels of NE were not significantly different regardless of whether they received regular group programming or intergenerational programming that day. However, a significant type of programming effect was seen in the *during* time period, t(14) 3.0, p < .01. Participants showed substantially less NE when working with children than when engaged in standard day-care activities at this time period. In fact, NE was rarely seen at all during intergenerational programming.

In summary, intergenerational programming produced substantially larger amounts of CE and smaller amounts of PE, AE, and NE than did regular day-care programming, as was hypothesized.

However, persons working with children did not show any generalization or maintenance of this effect outside of the intergenerational programming context.

Effects on Affect

We had originally hypothesized that participation in Montessori-based intergenerational programming would be associated with higher levels of positive affect (pleasure) and lower levels of negative affect (anxiety/fear and sadness) than participation in regular adult day-care programming. This was partially confirmed.

Pleasure. With regard to pleasure, significant main effects were found for type of programming, $F(1,13) = 39.5$, $p < .001$, and time of observation, $F(2,26) = 13.7$, $p < .001$. However, these main effects were mitigated due to the presence of a significant Type of Programming x Time of Observation interaction, $F(2,26) = 25.7$, $p < .001$. Means and standard deviations associated with this interaction are also shown in Table 9.2.

With regard to type of programming, similar amounts of pleasure were observed in the before and after time periods, regardless of whether or not participants worked with children or took part in regular day-center programming that day. This was followed by intergenerational or control programming. However, a significant type of programming effect was seen in the *during* time period, $t(14) = 7.1$, $p < .001$. Participants showed substantially more pleasure when working with children than when engaged in standard day-care activities at this time period.

Anxiety/Fear. With regard to anxiety/fear, a significant interaction was found for Group x Type of Programming was found, $F(1,13) = 9.7$, $p < .008$. Participants in Group 1 showed a slight decrease in overall anxiety/fear during the study phase in which they worked with children, $M = 1.0$ ($SD = 0.02$), compared to the study phase when they were not working with children, $M = 1.3$ ($SD = 0.3$). However, for participants in Group 2, a slightly higher overall level of anxiety/fear was seen in the study phase in which they worked with children, $M = 1.2$ ($SD = 0.2$), compared to the study phase when they were not working with children, $M = 1.1$ ($SD = 0.1$). Within each group, a paired *t*-test for the type of programming effect approached significance ($p < .05$). It is important to note that

TABLE 9.2   Means (and *SD*s) of Observed Pleasure Ratings as a Function of Type of Programming and Time of Observation

Time of Observation	Type of Programming	
	Montessori-Based Intergenerational	Regular Programming
Before	1.74 (0.4)	1.69 (0.4)
During	2.48 (0.5)	1.49 (0.3)
After	1.60 (0.4)	1.51 (0.3)

anxiety/fear was rarely displayed under any conditions, and that the changes we found in our measure of anxiety/fear may not be clinically meaningful in these data.

Sadness. No significant effects were found for sadness. It was rarely observed in this setting under any circumstances.

In summary, our Montessori-based intergenerational program produced significantly higher levels of pleasure than did standard day-center programming, but these effects did not generalize outside of the time frame in which participants were actually in contact with children. This pattern parallels effects found for our engagement measures. No such pattern emerged for measures of negative affect, primarily because ratings indicated that anxiety/fear and sadness were rarely seen in participants under any circumstances. Given that the day center had a reputation as providing a wide variety of high quality activities programming, this is not surprising.

CONCLUSIONS

From a qualitative standpoint, older adults and preschool children seemed to enjoy taking part in Montessori-based intergenerational programming. As we had observed in our pilot study, children viewed taking part in this program as a special event, and we had to take pains to make sure that all of the children taking part had equal access to our older adults. Adult day center clients looked forward to working with children and would ask staff members if the children were coming when seeing research staff members in the center.

In general, our hypotheses regarding quantitative outcomes were confirmed. Adult day-care clients, when working with children, showed more CE and pleasure and less PE, AE, and NE, than when taking part in regular adult day care activities. Another clear pattern that emerged was that the effects of intergenerational programming were generally limited to times when adult day-care clients were in direct contact with children. In other words, we did not see evidence of a "carry over" effect in these same participants at other times of the day.

Some persons might question the usefulness of an intergenerational program or any intervention for persons with dementia that only produces effects when the intervention is being applied. We have two responses to this perspective. First, the creation of higher quality engagement in persons with dementia is highly desirable under any circumstances. Expecting an effect when a psychosocial intervention is not being applied may not be reasonable in persons with declarative memory deficits. This is especially true when such individuals are extremely reactive to their immediate environments, as is often the case with persons with dementia. Psychosocial interventions for persons with dementia generally will not perform like a pharmacological agent within a biological system. Second, perhaps the better question is, "How can we provide more opportunities for persons with dementia to encounter interventions that produce high quality and quantity of engagement during the course of their daily routines?" When we can offer more opportunities to persons with dementia to take part in intergenerational programming as developed in this study at other times of the day, and/or other activities that effectively engage these persons, we will see more high quality engagement and positive affect throughout their day (see Camp, Cohen-Mansfield, & Capezuti, 2002).

In addition, it should be remembered that the effects produced by our program were found in a setting noted for its good quality and variety of activities. In addition, adult day-center clients are still capable of being maintained in the community. Effects produced by Montessori-based intergenerational programming may be larger in other settings, such as long-term care facilities. We are currently analyzing data from our program gathered in a long-term care setting. Finally, we are currently developing ways to expand intergenerational programming and to make it more available to persons with dementia in real-world contexts. For example, we are developing group activities in which an older adult with dementia is partnered with a preschool child as a team. Multiple teams then take part in games utilizing Montessori-based principles (e.g., use of procedural memory, motor learning, use of external cues with self-correction, etc.). We are creating training materials to enable staff at multiple facilities to implement such programming. It is our hope that effective intergenerational programming for persons with dementia will become more available in the future and that it will be part of an overall trend to provide more meaningful and engaging activities for these individuals.

ACKNOWLEDGMENT

This research was supported by grant # R21 MH5785 from the National Institute of Mental Health (NIMH) to Dr. Camp. Questions and correspondence regarding this manuscript should be submitted to: Cameron J. Camp, PhD, Meyers Research Institute, 27100 Cedar Road, Beachwood, OH 44122. (216) 839-6632; e-mail ccamp@myersri.com.

REFERENCES

Acello, B. (1997, March). Managing difficult behavior. *Journal of Nursing Assistants, 24–26.*

Alzheimer's Association (1995). *Activity programming for persons with dementia: A sourcebook.* Chicago: Alzheimer's Association.

Angelis, J. (1990). Bringing old and young together. *Vocational Education Journal, 65*(1), 19–21.

Aronstein, A., Olsen, R., & Schulman, E. (1996). The nursing assistants use of recreational interventions for behavioral management of residents with Alzheimer's disease. *American Journal of Alzheimer's Disease, 11*(3), 26–31.

Beck, C., Zgola, J., & Shue, V. (2000). Activities of daily living: An essential component of programming for persons with Alzheimer's disease. *Alzheimer's Care Quarterly, 1*(2), 46–55.

Bowlby, C. (1993). *Therapeutic activities with persons disabled by Alzheimer's disease and related disorders.* Gaithursburg, MD: Aspen.

Buettner, L. (1999). Simple pleasures: A multilevel sensorimotor intervention for nursing home residents with dementia. *American Journal of Alzheimer's Disease, 14*(1), 41–52.

Buettner, L. L, Lundegren, H., Lago, D., Farrell, P., & Smith, R. (1996).

Therapeutic recreation as an intervention for persons with dementia and agitation. *American Journal of Alzheimer's Disease, 11*(5), 4–12.

Camp, C. J. (1999). *Montessori-based activities for persons with dementia (vol.1).* Myers Research Institute, Menorah Park Center for Senior Living.

Camp, C. J., Cohen-Mansfield, J., & Capezuti, E. A., (2002). Use of non-pharmacologic interventions among nursing home residents with dementia. *Psychiatric Services, 53*(11), 1397–1401.

Camp, C. J., Judge, K. S., Bye, C. A., Fox, K. M., Bowden, J., Bell, M., et al (1997). An intergenerational program for persons with dementia using Montessori methods. *The Gerontologist, 37*(5), 688–692.

Camp, C. J, Koss, E,, & Judge, K. S. (1999). Cognitive assessment in late stage dementia. In P. A. Lictenberg (Ed.), *Handbook of assessment in clinical gerontology* (pp. 442–467). New York: John Wiley & Sons.

Dawson, P., Wells, D. L., & Kline, K. (1993). *Enhancing the abilities of persons with Alzheimer's and related dementias.* New York: Springer Publishing.

Dellmann-Jenkins, M. (1997). A senior-centered model of intergenerational programming with young children. *The Journal of Applied Gerontology, 16*(4), 495–506.

Dellmann-Jenkins, M., Lambert, D., & Fruit, D. (1991). Fostering preschoolers' prosocial behaviors toward the elderly: The effect of an intergenerational program. *Educational Gerontology, 17*(1), 21–32.

Dreher, B. (1997). Montessori and Alzheimer's: A partnership that works. *American Journal of Alzheimer's Disease, 12*(3), 138–140.

Fazio, S., Chavin, M., & Clair, A. A. (1999). Activity based Alzheimer care: A national training program. *American Journal of Alzheimer's Disease, 14*(3), 149–156.

Folstein, M. F., Folstein, S. E., & McHugh, P. R. (1975). "Mini-Mental State": A practical method for grading the cognitive state of patients for the clinician. *Journal of Psychiatric Rehabilitation, 12*(3), 189–198.

Griff, M., Lambert, D., Dellmann-Jenkins, M., & Fruit, D. (1996). Intergenerational activity analysis with three groups of older adults: Frail, community-living, and Alzheimer's. *Educational Gerontology, 22*(6), 601–612.

Hellen, C. (1998). *Alzheimer's disease: Activity-focused care.* Boston: Butterworth-Heinemann.

Judge, K. S., Camp, C. J., & Orsulic-Jeras, S. (2000). Use of Montessori-based activities for clients with dementia in adult day care: Effects on engagement. *American Journal of Alzheimer's Disease, 15*(1), 42–46.

Kocarnik, R. A., & Ponzetti, J. J. (1986). The influence of intergenerational contact on child care participants' attitudes toward the elderly. *Child Care Quarterly, 15*(4), 244–250.

Laurenhue, K. (2000). Broadening horizons: Activities with people with dementia. *Alzheimer's Care Quarterly, 1*(2), 38–45.

Lawton, M. P., Van Haitsma, K., & Klapper, J. (1996). Observed affect in nursing home residents with Alzheimer's disease. *Journal of Gerontology, 51B*(1), P3–P14.

Lawton, M. P., Van Haitsma, K., Perkinson, M., & Ruckdeschel, K. (1999). Observed affect and quality of life in dementia: Further affirmations and problems. *Journal of Mental Health and Aging, 5*(1), 69–81.

Newman, S., & Ward, C. (1992–1993). An observational study of intergenerational activities and behavior change in dementing elders at adult day care centers. *International Journal of Aging and Human Development, 36*(4), 321–333.

Orsulic-Jeras, S., Judge, K. S., & Camp, C. J. (2000). Montessori-based activities for long-term care residents with advanced dementia: Effects on engagement and affect. *The Gerontologist, 40*(1), 107–111.

Orsulic-Jeras, S., Schneider, N. M., & Camp, C. J. (2000). Montessori-based activities for long-term care residents with dementia. *Topics in Geriatric Rehabilitation, 16*(1), 78–91.

Orsulic-Jeras, S., Schneider, N. M., Camp, C. J., Nicholson, P., & Helbig, M. (2001). Montessori-based dementia activities in long-term care: Training and implementation. *Activities, Adaptation, and Aging, 25*(314), 107–120.

Plautz, R. E., & Camp, C. J. (2001). Activities as agents for intervention and rehabilitation in long-term care. In B. R. Bonder & M. B. Wagner (Eds.), *Functional performance in older adults* (2nd ed., pp. 405–425). Philadelphia: F. A. Davis.

Short-Degraff, M. A. & Diamond, K. (1996). Intergenerational program effects on social responses of elderly adult day care members. *Educational Gerontology, 22*(5), 467–482.

Squire, L. R. (1992). Memory and the hippocampus: A synthesis from findings with rats, monkeys, and humans. *Psychological Review, 99*(2), 195–231.

Squire, L. R. (1994). Declarative and nondeclarative memory: Multiple brain system supporting learning and memory. In D. L. Schacter & E. Tulving (Eds.), *Memory systems 1994* (pp. 203–232). Cambridge, MA: MIT Press.

Stevens, A. B., Camp, C. J., King, C. A., Bailey, E. H., & Hsu, C. (1998). Effects of a staff implemented therapeutic group activity for adult day care clients. *Aging and Mental Health, 2*(4), 333–342.

Stevens, A. B., King, C. A., & Camp, C. J. (1993). Improving prose memory and social interaction using question asking reading with adult day care clients. *Educational Gerontology, 19*(7), 651–662.

Vance, D., Camp, C.J., Kabacoff, M., & Greenwalt, L. (1996). Montessori methods: Innovative interventions for adults with Alzheimer's disease. *Montessori Life, 8*(1), 10–12.

Volicer, L., & Bloom-Charette, L. (1999). *Enhancing the quality of life in advanced dementia.* Boston: University School of Medicine.

Ward, C. R., Los Kamp, L., & Newman, S. (1996). The effects of participation in an intergenerational program on the behavior of residents with dementia. *Activities, Adaptation, and Aging, 20*(4), 61–76.

Zgola, J. (1987). *Doing things: A guide to programming activities for persons with Alzheimer's disease and related disorders.* Baltimore: Johns Hopkins University Press.

CHAPTER 10

Using a Learning Environment to Promote Intergenerational Relationships and Successful Aging

Catherine Whitehouse, Stephanie J. FallCreek, and Peter J. Whitehouse

Intergenerational health is an emerging multifaceted concept (Wadsworth & Whitehouse, 2001). It may incorporate system-level issues about allocation of health resources (equity and sustainability), as well as individual level issues (knowledge, attitudes, and skills) among different generations. In this chapter, we explore some of the facets of intergenerational health in the context of a collaboration between two community organizations, the Intergenerational School (focused on multiage education) and Fairhill Center (focused on successful aging), as they cocreate a relationship to nurture life-span learning as one important foundation for health.

INTERGENERATIONAL HEALTH

Our approach recognizes health as both a state of being and a resource that may be possessed and used by individuals, families, and communities. One classic definition of health is "a state of complete physical, social, and mental well being, and not merely the absence of disease or infirmity" (World Health Organization, 1948). This implies that good health as a "state of being" is an end in itself—something to be pursued for its own sake. We agree—just as knowledge may be pursued "for its own sake" as well as for an instrumental purpose. In addition, we also suggest that good health (individual, community, and/or intergenerational)—is equally important as a resource that may be used to enhance the prospects for leading a personally satisfying and socially purposeful life throughout one's life span. Both of these aspects of intergenerational health are in harmony with our efforts to nurture intergenerational relationships in a variety of shared learning environments.

As the overall theme of this book suggests, one critical resource for successful aging is health and wellness throughout the life span. Whether "state of being" or resource, for most people, personal health exists in a dynamic relationship with our natural and built environments and with people of other generations—most immediately with family and others in the community. Particularly, we recognize that from infancy through end-of-life transitions, the health of each member in the multigenerational and extended family unit has the potential to influence the physical and psychosocial well-being of every other member.

Another aspect of intergenerational health is the implication that communities have a responsibility to create and promote health care systems that encourage lifelong healthy habits. Moreover, in terms of the resources needed for good health, if equity among generations and sustainability from generation to generation is not achieved, there is the potential for conflict between generations. In prehistoric times, it is likely that individuals who survived late into life shared knowledge of past problem-solving successes that promoted the survival of those small vulnerable communities. In modern times, so, too, do older people have the experiences (and tools) of a lifetime to share so that younger generations may thrive. One measure of intergenerational health in a community or society may be how effectively positive health values are transmitted from one generation to the next. These values should include commitments to environmental sustainability and commitment to the frail in our societies.

The fundamental method by which generational health is promoted at the level of the individual, family, or community is through education, formal and informal. Generations learning together historically seem to have been the manner in which cultural knowledge is transmitted. Yet, in our society, many earlier opportunities have been lost. High levels of geographic mobility have decreased the time available for sharing between different generations of the same family, especially grandparents and grandchildren. Residential age segregation in service delivery settings and the proliferation of diverse types of retirement communities further reduce the opportunities for day-to-day interaction between elder and younger people.

A recent task force (Cleveland Foundation, 2002) suggested at least three important lifestyle/life-skill resources to facilitate successful aging. These included the following:

- adapting effectively to life's inevitable changes and challenges,
- cultivating and sustaining dynamic relationships, and
- living with a sense of purpose and joy.

Personal health is a platform upon which to build, or a resource that may be used as people seek to live and age in a way that nurtures a sense of well-being. Intergenerational health in this context means shared learning (knowledge, attitudes, values and skills) among and between generations so that people of all ages prepare for their own successful aging and that of others around them.

This depends upon both a life span and an intergenerational approach. While simultaneously respecting personal autonomy, the interdependence of the generations as well as the interdependence of individuals in the shared social, natural, and built environment is a core principle of this philosophy. It is not only beneficial but, perhaps, urgent, to develop models and strategies that reinvigorate intergenerational sharing and learning. We will describe one such model that is being developed through the collaboration between Fairhill Center and The Intergenerational School.

THE COLLABORATORS

Fairhill Center

Fairhill Center was created in 1988 when a social services agency (Benjamin Rose) and a large health care system (University Hospitals Health System, Inc.) came together with a vision for a collaborative campus of nonprofit organizations that shared, wholly or in part, a mission or service for older adults. The campus previously had served both as a Merchant Marine Hospital (1930–1953) and a state inpatient psychiatric facility (1956–1983). It is located in Cleveland on 10 acres and is composed of multiple buildings.

Fairhill Center, as an organization, has evolved over time to encompass two primary roles: facilitator of the collaborative campus of multiple organizations (i.e., property developer and landlord and relationship manager); and facilitator/provider of service programs in two areas: Wellness and Wisdom, and Care and Caregiving. The Intergenerational Resource Center, a Wellness and Wisdom program, was founded in 1994. It illustrates Fairhill's early recognition that fostering intergenerational relationships is one component of nurturing a successfully aging community. All Fairhill Center's service programs include educational aspects, and most emphasize education to promote self-care, self-help, and mutual support among peers. The Computer Learning Center, for example, provides training for 250–300 older persons annually, with instructors, marketing, administration, and coordination provided by peer volunteers.

Fairhill Center's mission statement: "Fairhill Center connects individuals, organizations, and choices to foster successful aging" highlights its facilitating and linking role. Its strategic plan focuses on completing renovation of the campus and leading the community in the creative recruitment and deployment of volunteers in all aspects of organizational service.

Origin of the Concept of the Intergenerational School

The concept of an intergenerational school emerged from conversations between Catherine and Peter Whitehouse (Whitehouse, Bendezu, FallCreek, & Whitehouse, 2000). Catherine Whitehouse has always been interested in the education of children, having trained in educational psychology and child development. She had served in several capacities as a psychologist and educator in both public and private schools. Peter Whitehouse has studied challenges to memory and learning imposed on people by conditions such as Alzheimer's disease. He was interested specifically in creating a learning environment that would facilitate persons with memory problems maintaining their cognitive vitality and contributions to community (Whitehouse, 2003). Moreover, Whitehouse felt that such an intergenerational learning community would contribute to environmental stewardship and community discussions about ethical issues (Whitehouse, 1999). These sets of interests converged while studying learning at different points of the life spectrum. Catherine Whitehouse's ambition to start a school based on her concepts of child development and educational pedagogy well matched the ideas emerging from Peter Whitehouse's work on experiential learning in older adults. The notion of housing The Intergenerational School at Fairhill Center emerged quickly.

The Collaborative Model

One of the authors of this chapter, Dr. Stephanie J. FallCreek, immediately was enthusiastic about the idea of an intergenerational school. The concepts of intergenerational learning and a welcoming attitude toward kinship care families, were in complete harmony with Fairhill's approach to intergenerational community building, as well as with her own doctoral work in social exchange theory. She joined with the Whitehouses as a codeveloper of the school. After Board-level discussions at Fairhill, the three codevelopers decided that the Intergenerational School would be developed as an independent, nonprofit organization and campus tenant rather than as a program of the Fairhill Center. A strong degree of collaboration was anticipated, as the two organizations were highly mission-compatible and Fairhill provided a nurturing environment for the school during its organizational start-up period.

As of this writing, The Intergenerational School (TIS) has completed its third year of operation at Fairhill. Over that time, TIS has completed its planned expansion of students and space. In the 2003–2004 school year, TIS will educate approximately 100 Cleveland area schoolchildren and occupy two wings (about 7,000 square feet of space) in the heart of Fairhill Center. As the developers expected, during this time a variety of programs have been developed by TIS in collaboration with Fairhill Center and other organizations with the goal of promoting lifelong learning, a spirit of volunteerism, and community outreach.

The Intergenerational School: An Ohio Community School

The Intergenerational School opened its doors to learners of all ages on August 30 of 2000 in shared space with Fairhill Center's Intergenerational Resource Center. The Intergenerational School is an Ohio Community School. As such, TIS is a tuition-free independent public school, not a private or voucher school. The Intergenerational School is open to any resident of Cleveland or adjacent school districts. The school has nonselective admission and word of mouth has proven to be the major means of student recruitment. Like all Ohio Community Schools, TIS is offered as a public school choice to area residents.

The Intergenerational School receives funding from the State of Ohio of approximately $5,000 per student. This is considerably less than the funds available to surrounding public school systems that have the advantage of generating additional monies through local tax levies. As a public school, TIS is both academically and fiscally accountable to the State of Ohio.

Governed by its own board of directors, the Intergenerational School seeks to accomplish the goals articulated in its mission statement, which reads, "The Intergenerational School fosters an educational community of excellence that provides skills and experiences for lifelong learning and spirited citizenship for learners of all ages."

The Intergenerational School is educationally innovative in several respects (Whitehouse et al., 2000). First, it uses a developmental curriculum that includes four stages of learning growth. Rather than organize students into the more traditional but arbitrary age-based and age-segregated grade levels, students are clustered in flexible multiage groups based on developmental learning needs. Small class sizes of 16 students permit each child to learn in a way and at a pace individually tailored to that child's unique needs and capabilities. The progressive pedagogical framework promotes independence, student decision making, self-assessment, and a reflective stance toward learning. This is in sharp contrast to the highly regimented, scripted, one-size-fits-all pedagogies that seem to be making a resurgence in education today (Kohn, 2000; Ohanian, 1999). At TIS, many elements of the "one-room schoolhouse" are back.

The second key innovation is the infusion of intergenerational concepts and relationships into all areas of the curriculum. This infusion has several goals. Not only does it encourage students to form and value individual relationships across the life span, it also supports and complements the academic instruction taking place daily. In this chapter, we examine several of these programs in more detail: a reading mentor program intended to maximize literacy development through the sharing of children's literature, an intergenerational computer class that supported the technology and science curriculum, a partnering program with long-term care facilities that supported the social studies curriculum, and a school-based nursing education program that supports the wellness and health curriculum.

TIS INTERGENERATIONAL PROGRAMS
AND COLLABORATIONS

Reading Mentors

Literacy is at the core of the curriculum. An intergenerational children's literature collection that forms one component of an outstanding school library was developed through a variety of funding resources. This focus on literacy and literature is at the heart of the most longstanding and successful intergenerational program at TIS, involving reading mentors of a variety of ages (from local college students to retired seniors) and socioeconomic backgrounds (from residents of local affluent suburbs to residents of urban poverty areas). Reading mentors, who are specifically not "tutors," participate in a series of training workshops and then commit to at least 2 hours weekly of reading stories to and with students in a one-on-one setting. Mentor-student relationships developed over the sharing of such stories lead to a deepening respect for each other as well as a love of books and reading. Certainly these traits provide a firm foundation for high levels of reading achievement.

The reading mentor program has benefited from the experience of Fairhill's Intergenerational Resource Center, which also offers summer and after school intergenerational mentoring programs. Furthermore, literacy efforts also outreach to TIS families. Family members have been engaged as learners in the school from the very beginning, with educational programs offered to them on such topics as How Children Learn and Gun Safety.

Intergenerational Computer Learning:
The Lake Erie Project

Another area of experiential learning that is a priority for the school is in the area of technology, wherein intergenerational learning is a natural model. In our increasingly technological age, familiarity with and access to computer technology greatly enhances opportunities for lifelong learning. Fairhill Center already had a successful senior computer learning center that trained older adults in various computer uses. In the intergenerational computer class, older adults who were "graduates" of the Fairhill program, worked with children from the Intergenerational School on a science-based technology project. TIS students had been studying the ecosystem of Lake Erie in their classroom. Together, seniors and TIS students enriched this understanding by further investigating personally selected topics of interest through Internet research. Each senior/student then learned how to create a PowerPoint presentation to show the results of their research to the school body. Thus, the participants not only learned about computers, but also about the natural resources in their own environment.

Lest we think that the only, or even the most important outcome of this class was the knowledge of computers or about the ecosystem of Lake Erie, we might share the thoughts of David Rivelus, who was one of the senior participants:

> When I was invited to volunteer as a mentor, colearner at The Intergenerational School, I was not sure if I would be good at this assignment, due to my lack of experience working with children. The impression I had was that the students with whom I would come in contact would, in all probability, come from homes of unconcerned and poor parents. I believed the children would be lacking in the social graces, slovenly in appearance, and slow learners.
>
> When I arrived to class the first day in my sweats, I was in for a big surprise. My hallucination exploded! The children were well dressed, bright, eager to learn, extremely polite, and had outgoing personalities. They were a delight to be with, and they made me feel young and vibrant again. I made it a point from that time on to be sure that I, too, came well dressed to class.
>
> As for the parents, I had the opportunity of meeting some of them at a luncheon, and everyone with whom I came in contact were as deeply committed to their children's education as those of us from suburbia.

Long-Term Care Partners

Another area of intergenerational learning supported the social studies curriculum by connecting the students to residences of long-term care facilities in the immediate proximity of the school. Our initial program in this area took place at the Kethley House, a nursing home facility and a division of the Benjamin Rose Institute. It involved music therapy with students and residents with moderate to severe dementia participating. Over 3 years, this type of programming has expanded to include each TIS class being in a relationship with the residents of a long-term care facility.

Teachers are free to tailor the learning component of these programs to meet student needs and curricular goals, keeping in mind that the formation of intergenerational bonds and the sharing of stories is always at the core of the partnership. One such program took place at Menorah Park Center for Senior Living, and it involved sharing oral histories and stories with residents there using lesson plans based on the book *Wilfred Gordon McDonald Partridge,* by Mem Fox. This book describes a young boy who interacts with nursing-home residents to learn about the concept of memory and then shares mementoes and stories with an older lady who has a problem with her memory. The oral histories gathered from Menorah Park residents (assisted in some cases by their family members) formed the basis of the writing component of the project. The final result was a beautiful quilt describing the stories that the young students and the residents cocreated using objects to stimulate their discussions of past memories.

Younger TIS students participated in a project at the Kethley House where "manners" was the theme. Students interacted with residents and learned how to interview them about their life stories, to play bingo, and to interact socially at meals. The final tea party was an opportunity for five- and six-year-olds to demonstrate their learning about etiquette as well as show off their dress clothes to their senior partners.

Case Western Reserve University—Multigenerational Collaborations

The intergenerational learning projects at The Intergenerational School involved more than just the very old and the very young students in public school. Hence, the term "multigenerational" may be the most appropriate one to use when describing our programs.

The Intergenerational School has developed a variety of collaborations with Case Western Reserve University to involve undergraduates with both seniors and children. An initial collaboration involved AquaCorps, a division of the Corporation for National Service focusing on environmental studies. Undergraduates worked with students in our first summer-school program learning about the concept of the watershed and making a field trip to assess the quality of the water and the environment in Doan Creek, which is the major part of a nearby watershed.

Currently, we are actively developing a program with the faculty of the Frances Payne Bolton School of Nursing at Case Western Reserve University, in which undergraduate student nurses work with students and families from the school to learn about community-based health. This constitutes a service-learning component for the undergraduate nursing program and a training site for nursing students. It is hoped that, as this program grows, faculty-supervised student nurses will eventually provide family health screenings and prevention-oriented health education at a school-based site. The school also has served as a learning site for classes in the innovative Seminar Approach to General Education and Scholarship (SAGES) Program at Case Western Reserve University. Freshmen in seminars on the life of the mind and on wisdom visited the school. In Peter Whitehouse's course on wisdom, they developed learning modules to share some aspect of wisdom at a weekend wisdom carnival.

CONCLUSION

The concept of an intergenerational public school is unique. As far as we can tell, it is the only school of its kind. The development of such a school not only required the coming together of a variety of models of learning and people with various experiences from different educational settings; it also required a physical home, located in a welcoming community. The collaboration grew from beliefs and values common to the two organizations, namely that (1) engaging older people in community service both enhances the community and benefits the volunteer, and (2) aging needs to be viewed as a lifelong experience if successful and productive aging is to be the result. The presence of the Intergenerational School at Fairhill Center has strengthened the campus community. The problem of incorporating young, boisterous learners in an environment that otherwise includes research, education, administrative work, and activities programs for older people and families proved to be far easier than anticipated. The young students offer a vitality to the environment that is derived from their youthful exuberance. The setting offers the opportunity for students to appreciate that they are a part of a larger community in which they can learn about older people who are living and learning in a community with a diversity of other programs.

The Intergenerational School is viewed as programmatically effective by one of its primary and earliest funders, the Cleveland Foundation. The Cleveland Foundation also has sponsored an evaluation study of the Intergenerational School and other Cleveland community schools that is being done by Western Michigan University (WMU) Evaluation Center. WMU has consistently praised the educational and organizational operations of TIS. Similarly, the school is viewed as a model of success educationally and in terms of its financial accountability by both the auditors and evaluators from the State of Ohio. These accomplishments are undoubtedly due to the quality leadership of administrative staff and teachers, working in close harmony with the commitments of students and parents. They also no doubt relate to the contributions that Fairhill Center makes in providing a welcoming intergenerational home for the school that facilitates reaching out not only to other campus organizations but also to other community organizations such as Case Western Reserve University. A campus such as Fairhill, which blends medical and social models of service with the spirit of nonprofit volunteerism, represents an innovative approach to enhancing the prospects for successful aging in the community.

When collaborative intergenerational programs are vehicles for the exchange of resources and learning among older and younger generations for individual and community benefit, the fabric of our community is woven more durably and brightly. Intergenerational conversations, stories, and experiences can create a climate of respect and mutuality that knows no age limits. The students (old and young alike) of TIS are well prepared to transcend the generational and situational boundaries that too often inhibit our planning and policy. If successful aging requires adapting to the changes and challenges of aging, these students have witnessed and experienced the benefits of a lifelong learning approach to problem solving. If successful aging requires the cultivation of dynamic relationships, these students have practiced caring and sharing and care across the generations as well as in the classroom. If successful aging requires living with a sense of purpose and joy, then these spirited intergenerational partners are becoming well-versed in service learning as a joyful example. It is our intent and belief that the Intergenerational School, as an innovative approach to public education, will prepare its graduates to influence the larger community with the knowledge, skills, and values needed to promote and model lifelong learning, intergenerational health, and successful aging wherever life may lead them.

ACKNOWLEDGMENTS

We would like to thank Mr. Mark Elliott, the chairman of the board of The Intergenerational School; Mr. James Wallace, Treasurer and Coordinator of the Computer Learning Center of Fairhill Center; and Mr. David Revelis, a volunteer at The Intergenerational School and Fairhill Center, for their contributions to the seminar upon which this chapter is based.

REFERENCES

Cleveland Foundation. (2002). *Successful aging initiative.* [Electronic version] Retrieved December 27, 2002, from www.successfulaging.org

Kohn, A. (2000). *The schools our children deserve: Moving beyond traditional classes and "tougher standards."* Boston: Mariner Books, Houghton Mifflin.

Ohanian, S. (1999). *One size fits few.* Portsmouth, NH: Heinemann.

Wadsworth, N., & Whitehouse, P. J. (2001). Future of intergenerational programs. In M. D. Mezey, (Ed.), *The encyclopedia of elder care: The comprehensive resource on geriatric and social care* (p. 387). New York: Springer Publishing.

Whitehouse, P. J. (1999). The ecomedical disconnection syndrome. *Hastings Center Report, 29*(1), 41–44.

Whitehouse, P. J., Bendezu, E., FallCreek, S., & Whitehouse, C. (2000). Intergenerational community schools: A new practice for a new time. *Educational Gerontolology, 26,* 761–770.

Whitehouse, P. J. (2003). Paying attention to acetylcholine: The key to cognitive enhancement. In L. Descarries, K. Krnjevic, & M. Steriade (Eds.), *Progress in brain research* (pp. 311–317). The Netherlands: Elsevier Science.

World Health Organization. (1948). *Constitution.* Retrieved February 15, 2003, from http://policy.who.int/cgi-bin/om_isapi.dll?hitsperheading+on&infobase=basicdoc&record={9D5}&softpage=Docment4

Just Aging:
Issues in Intergenerational Health

Peter J. Whitehouse

Aging is about change. All living creatures age and, in fact, the universe ages as well. Aging as an idea is malleable. As a socially constructed label, the concept of aging has and will continue to evolve. How we envision our aging through time—in our academic work and in our lives—will create our futures as we evolve biologically and culturally.

This book and the conference upon which it was based were designed to enrich our thinking and enliven our passions about aging both as persons and as professionals. Although global in scope, the Cleveland region is our special focus. Our conference was held on October 13, 2002 just before The Cleveland Foundation launched its Successful Aging Initiative at its own conference on October 21. This initiative was based on the recognition that the Cleveland region has one of the oldest populations outside the Sunbelt and was designed to improve the opportunity for aging successfully. This chapter links both October events and offers a personal view of the lessons learned from these and subsequent events. It concludes by outlining some examples of new innovative community programs for all aging individuals—in other words, all of us.

Both our Case Western Reserve University (Case) Center for Aging and Health and the Cleveland Foundation conferences featured the concept of successful aging. As Moody (in this volume) points out in his chapter, this is an old concept much celebrated as part of

189

the creation of the "new gerontology." The term has been used in different ways, including either growing old without disease and dysfunction or adapting well to the limits and challenges associated with the aging process. "Productive aging" (see Morrow-Howell, p. 19) is an alternative term that brings necessary focus to the relationships between individual and society. However, each has a somewhat materialistic—even an economic—flavor to it. Terms like "conscious aging" allow opportunities to consider personal developmental and spiritual aspects of aging. An aspect of conscious aging is to face the inevitability of death in association with reexamining life's purpose nearer to its end.

The Task Force on Successful Aging of the Cleveland Foundation and many others have struggled with finding an appropriate-term to label aging (FallCreek, personal communication, 2003). In this epilogue, I also was challenged to find another modifier for aging. In keeping with Moody's focus on global ecological matters, I considered the term "natural aging." All life ages and, therefore, aging is natural. Clearly, as we consider the future of older persons in an over-populated world, the ever increasing damage to our ecosystems becomes paramount. The death of younger adults around the world and in Cleveland due to HIV/AIDS and violence leads to tremendous burdens on older adults in career and family life. However, I decided to modify the word "aging" with the word "just,"—that is, "just aging." Aging is so ubiquitous as a phenomenon and is present at least in the background in many conversations about life. Perhaps it needs no modifier. It is just aging. The use of this modifying term should not result in older people or their health care professionals assuming that all health conditions associated with growing older are caused by the aging process alone, however. Older people do suffer from diseases, although separating disease from normal age-related changes is not easy. For example, as we discuss later, the boundaries between age-related memory loss and Alzheimer's disease (AD) are unclear. Is AD really "just" aging or not? (Whitehouse, 2003).

However, I intend the word just in another sense, namely, to refer to justice. Here, our responsibility not only for our own lives and for those of our fellow living creatures, but for those who will come in the future becomes apparent. Thus, this title allows us to include our sense of responsibility for environmental stewardship and intergenerational equity. How can we in the United States consider successful aging and technologies such as life extension without considering people in other countries or many even in our own who have their aging process cut short by dying in childhood? How should we think of our use of natural resources in order to preserve them for future generations? Can the idea of an eco-economy or natural capitalism help make an unsustainable global capitalism more responsible? Can multinational pharmaceutical companies adjust to their priorities to be committed to a healthy world? To return to our example of AD, How much money should be spent on biological fixes when maintaining cognitive vitality as we age is much more than a medical problem?

We begin by reviewing what can be found in this book and what cannot be found. For example, a few topics were included in the conference but not in the book. We then use the issue of maintaining and enhancing cognitive vitality to illustrate some of the challenges to just aging. Finally, we end by describing selected ongoing activities in the Cleveland organizations that we hope will contribute to successful aging of our communities and their members.

FRAMING THE ISSUES GLOBALLY

Our book focuses on programs being developed in Cleveland and in Northeast Ohio. Yet, we examine these activities within a global conceptual framework. In our conferences, we did not focus on other countries struggling with similar aging issues. The world is aging most dramatically in countries that are perhaps less well able to adapt to changing demographics than are those in the West. Different cultural beliefs about aging will modify the range of possible societal responses to the growing number of older people in different countries. Perhaps, in fact, technologically advanced countries may not fare as well as those societies that respect the elderly and have a greater sense of intergenerational responsibility. Perhaps those societies will adjust better to the aging of our world.

One case example is Japan. This country has the longest life expectancy and one of the lowest birth rates. We can see in Japan perhaps most visibly the dynamic tension between the cultural attitudes of honoring the elderly and the challenges of providing care. Major changes are underway in the structure of the Japanese family, society, and economy to accommodate to this challenge. Fundamental rethinking about the notion of economic growth is part of this cultural debate. The implementation of the new national long-term care insurance system is enlivening debates about self-determination, changing attitudes about responsibility of care for family members and others, and creating debate about economic development focusing on sustainability rather than growth. Certain technological innovations—for example, the use of robots to care for bedridden elderly—are emerging in Japan. In Cleveland, our efforts are more advanced in the use of interactive technologies to support older people and their caregivers.

DEALING WITH DEATH

It is unfortunate that one of the sessions that was held in our Center for Aging and Health (CAH) conference was not represented in this book: a discussion of the care of the dying in hospice. Our attitudes toward death in general and to our own personal mortality dramatically affect our conceptions of our own aging and its successes and failures. Incorporating some conception of a successful death into our life stories is key. Health concerns at the end of life need to focus not just on extension of life but rather on the quality of life. Death is an important aspect of the quality of life. Addressing this issue often entails a religious or spiritual dimension. Mainstream religions as well as new emerging spiritual belief systems can dramatically affect our community's attitudes toward aging as well as to our own. In the Cleveland Foundation conference, the important work of the Center for Spiritual Eldering was featured. A commitment to preserving natural environments for their intrinsic beauty as well as because they are a necessity in supporting our own lives and those of future generations it seems an important part of a spiritual quest occurring later in life.

Although we do not address end-of-life care specifically in this book, we do address the impact of chronic disease on individuals and the long-term care system (Kahana, p. 101). Successful aging is dependent on preventing or adjusting to acute and chronic illnesses. We emphasize strongly in this book the importance of diet (Petot, p. 87) and exercise (Roberts, p. 71) and other changes in behavior to promoting a healthy long life. Age-related diseases will continue to challenge us as individuals and as a society attempting to provide a just distribution of health care resources. In this book, we emphasize the importance of the conception of intergenerational health. Although this is a new concept, it is based on the recognition that our own lives and the lives of our communities will be dramatically affected by how the generations work together to promote successful aging. Grandmothers raising grandchildren alone represent a growing population for Cleveland and elsewhere and are challenged by aging issues. The very old and the very young are the most frail members of our community. Just aging requires providing an appropriate balance between preventative wellness services for the young and long-term care for the elderly. Conversations about generational equity will likely intensify as health care resources become inadequate to keep up with the changing demographics of our population. At a societal level, the concept of intergenerational health provokes us to consider how to develop systems of care that allow different generations to contribute to each other's health in a reciprocal way. Reconceptualizing caregiving in the context of family (Musil et al., p. 143) and professions (DeGolia, p. 131) will be important. Valuing caregiving as a social, and even as an economic activity, and emphasizing the positive opportunities that come with caring will be essential.

INTERGENERATIONAL CONVERSATIONS

Intergenerational conversations create opportunities for learning. In fact, one might argue that improving health education is the most dramatic opportunity for improving the health of our nation and the world. Attempts to use Montessori methods to provide care for patients with dementia illustrate creative adaptation of educational approaches developed for one age to another (Camp, p. 159). The Intergenerational School also featured in this book (Whitehouse et al., p. 177) is an effort to create a more powerful learning environment that can enrich the lives of youngsters and oldsters alike. Many of its efforts contribute to intergenerational health directly and indirectly. A program with Case's School of Nursing allows these students to follow the health issues of urban school children and their families. The school participated in a national living dialogue (called Valeo) using an envisioning tool called Appreciative Inquiry to create positive conversations about health and to dream about and design healthier communities. The efforts to create an entirely new philosophy of education based around the conception of liberal education at Case are yet another example of efforts to promote lifelong learning. Cuyahoga Community College, the host of The Cleveland Foundation conference, has a wonderful track record of providing opportunities for older learners to contribute to the vitality of our Cleveland community through its Center for Applied Gerontology and other programs.

COGNITIVE VITALITY AND AD

The issue of cognitive vitality is critical to successful aging. As we age, our most vulnerable organ is the brain, and our greatest psychological concern is that of losing our mental faculties. Let us examine the role of preserving and enhancing cognition as a part of successful aging by focusing on the greatest fear of many, AD, and perhaps our greatest goal, the pursuit of wisdom.

The treatment of disease could be viewed as central to successful aging. How can one be a success as an older person if one is ill? Alzheimer's disease is one of the most common conditions affecting older people, causing significant stress to the affected person, his or her family, and society. The dominant approach to addressing the challenges of dementia is the biomedical model, which promises a cure in exchange for significant investment in basic biological research. An extrapolation of this viewpoint leads to the emerging interest in antiaging medicine and the quest of biogerontologists to find the fountain of youth. Rightly or wrongly, some responsible (and many irresponsible) individuals are contemplating the individual and societal consequences of developing a biological product that would actually slow or even arrest the aging process (Juengst et al, 2003). Scenarios are being created around the assumption that we could live, on average, 30 or more years beyond our expected life span. These future projections are based on incredible faith in scientific progress—which might be labeled "scientism,"—faith that such interventions are likely in the near-term future.

It is ironic that, in fact, in the last century, we have extended life expectancy by almost 30 years and are now beginning to see the consequence of changing demographics on the world's societies. We could learn lessons from the past 100 years to help us think about the next 100 years if we extend life through pills (Juengst et al, 2003). Clearly, much greater gain could be achieved in average life expectancy by focusing on basic issues of diet, exercise, and public health rather than on the potential for molecular biology and genetics to produce magic "silver" bullets.

Nevertheless, part of any successful aging initiative needs to address possible health and social system implications of the current claim that antiaging interventions are available. Individuals in this country spend perhaps $45 billion on so-called complementary and alternative health approaches. Many of these are directed toward life extension and cognitive enhancement. Theoretically, such products should not advertise themselves as treatments for diseases but rather for specific symptoms such as those people face as they age, such as memory problems.

AGING OR DISEASE?

A major issue for successful aging is, What constitutes a disease and what constitutes so-called normal aging? All of us face, even in midlife, the recognition that our cognitive abilities change with age. Challenges to multitasking and to short-term memory abound as we joke about senior moments. Yet, the dominant focus of our concerns about preserving cognitive vitality has been the avoidance of AD. AD is diagnosed by demonstrating progressive cognitive impairment associated with senile plaques and neurofibrillary tangles in the brain. Yet, where do age-related cognitive change and AD meet? It is a fuzzy boundary, one in which terms have been invented to characterize milder degrees of cognitive impairment such as aging associated memory impairment and mild cognitive impairment (Petersen et al., 2001; Whitehouse, 2003; Whitehouse, 2003; Whitehouse et al., 2000). The politics of science and medicine have led to the position that AD is not normal aging. This statement created expectations that a cure of the disease is possible in exchange for intense investment in biological science. Yet, clinicians recognize the challenges of separating the effects of age from this so-called disease. Does the label mild cognitive impairment as recommended by the American Academy of Neurology represent early AD, the absence of AD, or the inevitability of AD (Petersen et al., 2001)?

If we were to accept a certain degree of cognitive impairment as an expected part of aging, would our attitudes change? Could we compensate better both as individuals and as a society for cognitive changes as we all age? The focus on the fear of Alzheimer's disease has limited our ability to think of the possible intellectual growth opportunities as we age. Even though wisdom is not inevitable, longer life on this planet does create opportunities for the kind of experiences and reflections that could produce wisdom. Is not one goal of a successful and just aging the pursuit of individual and collective wisdom?

THE PURSUIT OF WISDOM

Wisdom is, ironically, a controversial term in our postenlightenment and postmodern society. It represents an ability to integrate thoughts and values often in the service of others in the practical matters of daily life. It includes with it a sense of humility and limits, as well as a profound sense of the mysteries of life. Throughout history, wisdom has served as a goal in many different cultural and religious traditions. Yet, in our society, particularly (and ironically) in our learning institutions, the pursuit of wisdom is viewed with ambivalence. One might expect that in the fields of psychology, ethics, and organizational behavior, we should attend to the question, What is wisdom and how can we enhance it? Yet, there is an embarrassment about wisdom, perhaps because of an ancient concept associated with foreign or less vital religious traditions. This model of wisdom focuses on the rarity of wisdom and posits that its pursuit represents arrogance. How ironic that as we talk about successful aging, we have distorted the opportunities for wisdom through our own lack of that trait.

In the view of this author, a better conception of wisdom is one that recognizes that we are wise to varying degrees and have the potential for attaining greater wisdom. Surely, we have a goal of education and of greater aging to enhance not only our own individual wisdom but the collective wisdom of our communities and our cultures. How else, in fact, can we address the enormously complex challenges that modern life presents? Just at such a time when we should be having our deepest conversations about wisdom, we have developed hostilities toward the kind of integrative thinking and feeling endeavor required to have a conversation about wisdom.

So, how do we go about enhancing cognitive vitality and, in fact, enhancing wisdom as we attempt to age successfully? Perhaps the answer lies in a pill. If AD is an extension of the normal age-related neurological changes that we all face, then perhaps the drugs for AD will help us all age with greater cognitive vitality. What if claimed preventatives for AD, such as antioxidants like vitamin E, in fact, arrest the process of normal brain aging? We have been exploring the ethics and practicalities of these kinds of approaches in our work in Cleveland. In collaboration with investigators at Stanford University, we have administered donepezil, the most widely prescribed medication for AD, to a group of 53-year-old pilots on a randomized double-blind controlled study (Yesavage et al., 2002). We compared the performance of these pilots on a placebo and on the active drug when asked to land a plane and handle emergencies in a flight simulator. In this realistic simulation of activities of daily living, which is predictive for actual performance in the skies, the pilots performed slightly better on donepezil than on the sugar pill. Can we imagine a day in which we will all be enhanced in our work and perhaps in our play by pharmacological means? Those of us who are coffee drinkers recognize the benefits of a mild cognitive boost in attention and arousal produced by that drug.

Yet, although pills may improve attention and perhaps how well we attend to life, they could affect our wisdom. It is unlikely that we should find wisdom in a pill. Moreover, it is probably not wise to imagine that antiaging research will lead to a neurological fountain of youth. What other alternatives do we have to create opportunities for the enhancement of collective wisdom? Perhaps opportunities lie in improving our educational efforts. As President Edward Hundert of Case claims—wisely, I think—that "educated learners love learning," but that "they love wisdom more." He is reinventing the concept of liberal education to transform our university. One key program is the program called Seminar Approach to General Education and Scholarship (SAGES). In our own work in SAGES, we developed a course on wisdom that included a service learning component. Case undergraduates developed a learning module to share with kindergartners through fourth graders in the Intergenerational School, some insight about wisdom. This one illustration is an attempt to create a learning environment in which to explore experiences that, we hope, might lead to some advancement in the intellectual and moral development of the learners. The challenges of creating learning spaces in which students of different ages can share and cocreate knowledge are great; the opportunities are greater. At the heart of creating learning spaces for growth in collective wisdom is the need to make available experiences and opportunities for reflection and storytelling. At the Intergenerational School, we include programming in computers and gardening, as well as reading that allows creating and sharing of stories. We are about to open an intergenerational playground that will celebrate the fact that learning is not all about work but is about play as well.

At the heart of attempts at intergenerational creation of wisdom lies the power of stories and the richness of narrative. At both the individual and community level, we will be successful to the extent that we can incorporate our individual stories with those of our friends and families. Our work with the Cleveland Foundation will focus on this narrative process as the heart of our work in lifelong learning and development (described below).

The chapter by Juengst (p. 13) represents the power of stories to draw us into the future. He imagines a future in which aging is valued more than youth. His creative literary product complements our other more scientific chapters (particularly Camp, p. 159) to build dialogues across generations. What is different perhaps between youth and old age is their proximity to the beginning and end of life. Clearly, a society in which older people are more valued needs to address the value of death in the life cycle, perhaps in relationship to its evolutionary and ecological necessity as well as to the anchoring of our mortality for our sense of purpose in life as well as to our vitality for living.

SUCCESSFUL AGING INITIATIVES—WHAT'S NEXT?

Based on the recommendations of their own task force and on some of the national leaders present at the October conference, the Cleveland Foundation launched their successful aging Initiatives in the fall of 2003. The creation of lifelong learning and development centers, opportunities for civic engagement, programs for career counseling, and interventions to make communities more elder friendly are the four components of the current program. Associated with this programming is a major public effort through educational television and other media to raise the visibility of the concept of successful aging in the region.

The first component to be launched is the lifelong learning and development centers. In collaboration with two other authors in this book, Stephanie FallCreek and Paul Alandt, we developed a successfully funded proposal entitled, 'What's Next?' The goal of our program, like the entire Cleveland Foundation initiative, is to create opportunities for individuals to age successfully. Our project involves three components. First, we assess individuals who are attracted to our program by using a variety of quantitative and qualitative methods focusing principally on the elaboration of their life stories. We used Appreciative Inquiry to celebrate and reflect on the most positive aspects of the individual's life in the past. We asked people to reflect about successful experiences in the area of knowledge and learning, health and wellness, beauty and aesthetics, and ethics and values. People are given unstructured opportunities to tell stories about when they felt the healthiest, the most energized by learning, the most profound sense of beauty, and the most authentic in living their values. After this assessment, people join us in a seminar series we call our core curriculum to share their stories and to further develop their sense of opportunities in these four domains of life. Our community partners include the Retired Senior Volunteers Program (RSVP), the Sophia Center of Ursuline College, and the Hospice of the Western Reserve. We are currently expanding our affiliated organizations to provide a rich panoply of learning and volunteering opportunities for our participants. Other courses will be offered through the Center for Spiritual Eldering as well as other opportunities for artistic expression and physical exercise. After completing the core curriculum, individuals will develop a plan to extend and enrich their life stories through a series of individual and community activities. The notions of individual development, civic engagement, and community learning are at the heart of both our concepts and programs, which are designed to enhance successful aging.

CONCLUSION

This book, the works of the authors in this book, and the two Cleveland conferences provide a foundation for our successful aging initiatives. Many other sources of information exist to assist the members of the Cleveland community in thinking about their own aging and the future of their community. We wish to think globally about such opportunities but to act locally in modifying our own behaviors and interactions with others to promote successful aging opportunities for all of us. Americans tend to celebrate autonomy and independence. Arguably, these are foundational principles for our country. Yet, the messages of the present and of our future are that we are all interdependent and that attention to the needs of our neighbors will ultimately give us the greatest degree of personal satisfaction. The world seems an increasingly uncertain place. It is far beyond the wisdom of any individual or group of individuals to understand fully all the challenges and opportunities that lie ahead. Nevertheless, it is in our individual life stories and their interactions with the stories of others that the grand narratives will play out their plots and themes, subplots, and subthemes. It is up to all of us to determine what's next.

REFERENCES

Camp, J. C., Lee, M. M., Orsulic-Jeras, S., & Judge, K. S. (2005). Effects of a Montessori-based intergenerational program on engagement and affect for adult day care clients with dementia. In M. L. Wykle, P. J. Whitehouse, & D. L. Morris (Ed.), *Successful aging through the life span.* New York: Springer Publishing.

DeGolia, P. A. (2005). Multigenerational issues that impact on successful aging in seniors caregiving. In M. L. Wykle, P. J. Whitehouse, & D.L. Morris (Ed.), *Successful aging through the life span.* New York: Springer Publishing.

Juengst, E. (2005). Can aging be interpreted as a healthy, positive process? In M. L. Wykle, P. J. Whitehouse, & D. L. Morris (Eds.), *Successful aging through the life span.* New York: Springer Publishing.

Juengst, E., Binstock, R. H., Mehlman, M., Post, S. G., & Whitehouse, P. J. (2003). Biogerontology, "Anti-aging medicine," and the challenges of human enhancement. *Hastings Center Report, 33*(4), 21–30.

Kahana, E., Kahana, B., Wisniewski, A., Bohne, A., King, C., Kercher, et al. (2005). Successful aging in the face of chronic disease. In M. L. Wykle, P. J. Whitehouse, & D.L. Morris (Eds.), *Successful aging through the life span.* New York: Springer Publishing.

Moody, H. R. (2005). From successful aging to conscious aging. In M. L. Wykle, P. J. Whitehouse, & D.L. Morris (Eds.), *Successful aging through the life span: Intergenerational issues in health.* New York: Springer Publishing.

Morrow-Howell, N., Tang, F., Kim, J., Lee, M., & Sherraden, M. (2005). Maximizing the productive engagement of older adults. In M. L. Wykle, P. J. Whitehouse, & D.L. Morris (Eds.), *Successful aging through the life span: Intergenerational issues in health.* New York: Springer Publishing.

Musil, C. M., Stoller, E. P., & Warner, C. B. (2005). Intergenerational caregiving in families: Structure, ethnicity, and building family ties. In M. L. Wykle, P. J. Whitehouse, & D.L. Morris (Ed.), *Successful aging through the life span.* New York: Springer Publishing.

Petersen, R. C., Stevens, J. C., Ganguli, M., Tangalos, E. G., Cummings, J. L., & DeKosky, S. T. (2001). Practice parameter: Early detection of dementia: Mild cognitive impairment (an evidence-based review) Report of the Quality Standards Subcommittee of the American Academy of Neurology. *Neurology, 56*(9), 1133–1142.

Petot, G. (2005). Food for thought . . . and good health. In M. L. Wykle, P. J. Whitehouse, & D.L. Morris (Ed.), *Successful aging through the life span*. New York: Springer Publishing.

Roberts, B. L., & Adler, P. (2005). Exercise and the generations. In M. L. Wykle, P. J. Whitehouse, & D. L. Morris (Ed.), *Successful aging through the life span*. New York: Springer Publishing.

Whitehouse, C., FallCreek, S., & Whitehouse, P. J. (2005). Using a learning environment to promote intergenerational relationships and successful aging. In M. L. Wykle, P. J. Whitehouse, & D. L. Morris (Eds.), *Successful aging through the life span*. New York: Springer Publishing.

Whitehouse, P. J. (2003). Mild Cognitive Impairment: The beginning of the end of AD. *Psychiatric Times.*

Whitehouse, P. J. (2003). Letter to Lancet "Classifications of the dementias," commentary on he Dementias article by Richie and Lovestone, *Lancet* 2002, 1759–1766. *Lancet, 361,* 1227.

Whitehouse, P. J., Maurer, K., & Ballenger, J. (Eds.). (2000). *Concepts of Alzheimer's disease: Biological, clinical, and cultural perspectives*. Baltimore: Johns Hopkins Press.

Yesavage, J. A., Mumenthaler, M. S., Taylor, J. L., Friedman, L., O'Hara, R., Sheikh, J., et al. (2002). Donepezil and flight simulator performance: Effects on retention of complex skills. *Neurology, 59*(1), 123–125.

Index

Springer Publishing Company

Gerotechnology
Research and Practice in Technology and Aging

David C. Burdick, PhD and
Sunkyo Kwon, PhD, Dipl-Psych, Editors

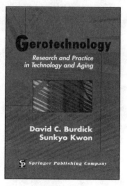

From the basics of gerotechnology—person-environment fit—to the core activity fields—computer and assistive devices and their applications—to prototypes for technical development and its application to everyday life, this volume explores the intersections of technology with aging and serves as both a primer and reference for educators, students, researchers, and practitioners.

Partial Contents:

Part I: Basic Aspects of Gerotechnology

- Technology in Everyday Life for Older Adults, *W. Rogers, C. Mayhom, and A. Fisk*
- Perceptual Aspects of Gerotechnology, *C. Scialfa, G. Ho, and J. Laberge*
- Aging and Technology: Social Science Approaches, *H. Mollenkopf*

Part II: Computers, Older Adults and Caregivers

- Why Older Adults Use or Do Not Use the Internet, *R. Morrell, C. Mayhorn, and K. Echt*
- Educational Tools for Web Designers, Older Adults and Caregivers, *A. Benbow*
- Computer-Mediated Communication and Its Use in Support Groups for Family Caregivers, *K. Smyth and S. Kwon*

Part III: Assistive Technology, Home and Environment

- Monitoring Household Occupant Behaviors to Enhance Safety and Well-Being, *D. Kutzik and A. Glascock*
- Technologies to Facilitate Health and Independent Living in Elderly Populations, *B. Tran*

Part IV: Models, Prototypes, and Specific Applications of Gerotechnology

- Driving Simulation and Older Adults, *G. Rebok and P. Keyl*

Part V: Cautions, Integration and Synthesis

- Ethical Realities: The Old, the New, and the Virtual, *G. Lesnoff-Caravaglia*

2005   320pp   0-8261-2516-6   hard $48.95 (outside US $53.80)

11 West 42nd Street, New York, NY 10036-8002 • Fax: 212-941-7842
Order Toll-Free: 877-687-7476 • Order On-line: www.springerpub.com